AF872683

Calming The Cancer Chaos

An Oncologist's Guide for Women to Understand, Organize, and Take Control of Their Cancer Care

Praise for *Calming The Cancer Chaos*

Our uniqueness—in goals, desires, fears, needs, values, and responsibilities—is amplified when confronting a life crisis, such as a severe illness. Furthermore, we often must make major decisions quickly, decisions that are right for us as well as people who depend upon us. Good decisions require information that is accurate, comprehensive, and tailored to our individuality. Dr. Tiffany Troso-Sandoval is a knowledgeable, insightful, and deeply caring physician with whom I have had the pleasure of working for many years. With this book in hand, a woman dealing with cancer would have the benefit of a truly trustworthy, experienced, and compassionate friend.

—Larry Norton, MD
Memorial Sloan Kettering's Norna S. Sarofim Chair, Senior Vice President in the Office of the President, Medical Director of the Evelyn H. Lauder Breast Center, and Deputy Cancer Center Director for Clinical and Translational Science, Former President of the American Society of Clinical Oncology, and BCRF Founding Scientific Director.

Calming the Cancer Chaos is not a book like so many others addressing the how, what, and when of a breast cancer diagnosis. It is a companion that takes all the hundreds and thousands of pieces of information given to the patient by their health care provider, navigator, family, friends, internet, chat rooms, survivors, and advocates and beautifully sifts through what is relevant vs not for that individual patient. No two patients will have the same journey. Empowering that individual patient to memorialize the information relevant to them allows the fears, confusion, and excessive noise to be streamlined into a document, a safe, honest place to navigate their own experience, revisit and actively participate in the course of their own journey. I have been privileged to care for thousands of patients diagnosed with early and advanced breast cancer over several decades. I have been on the other side of the desk, supporting family and friends through their own frightening diagnosis. At some point, the patient is left alone with the events of the day weighing on them. Dr. Troso-Sandoval has gifted the patient with a way to organize, document, and question in their workbook how to calmly confront what they will encounter tomorrow. I am excited that I have a novel book source with a much-needed workbook to offer my patients, allowing my voice to be heard and listened to, as needed, and creating a pathway for the patient's voice to be heard and listened to. Congratulations to Dr. Troso-Sandoval for her voice, as she has not only heard but listened to her patients over the years with compassion and understanding.

—Maria Theodoulou, MD
Program Director, Breast Cancer Medicine
New York Oncology Hematology
Former Attending Physician, Breast Medicine
Memorial Sloan Kettering Cancer Center, NYC
Professor of Medicine
Weill Cornell Graduate School of Medical Sciences

Congratulations to Dr. Troso-Sandoval, a talented oncologist whose approach is based on humanism, for providing this very practical, empowering guide that aims to bring the basics of breast cancer to the people who need to understand it quickly: people diagnosed and those who support them. This book teaches people with breast cancer, and other types as well, how to manage the medical, emotional, and logistical challenges of cancer—turning an overwhelming experience into a structured and more manageable journey. I often tell people: you never trained in cancer medicine, so I understand why it's overwhelming. This book fits squarely in the space of providing knowledge where it is necessary and moves all forward to self-advocacy where one's goals and preferences can marry the best approaches to breast cancer.

—Don Dizon, MD, FACP, FASCO
System Chief of Hematology Oncology, Cancer Service Line
Jane F. Desforges, MD, Chair in Hematology and Oncology, Tufts
University School of Medicine

Calming the Cancer Chaos delivers the information patients and caregivers need—clear, reliable guidance on diagnosis, treatment, and survivorship. With a remarkable combination of empathy and expertise, Dr. Tiffany Troso-Sandoval demystifies scans, grading, and staging—replacing fear and confusion with understanding. A vital guide I'll be recommending to patients, caregivers, loved ones, and advocates.

—Rebecca Bloom
Author of *When Women Get Sick: An Empowering Approach for Getting the Support You Need*

As a breast cancer survivor, this book really spoke to me. Cancer is chaos, plain and simple. One minute you're living your normal life, and the next you're drowning in appointments, scans, medical terms, and fear you never knew existed. Reading this, I kept thinking, *where was this when I was diagnosed*? What I love most is that it doesn't just throw information at you. It helps you make sense of it. It helps you organize it. And most importantly, it helps you feel a little less powerless in a situation that can make you feel completely out of control. Looking back, I know I spent so much time overwhelmed, scared, and just trying to keep up. A resource like this would have helped me slow down, understand what was happening, and advocate for myself better.

This isn't just a book—it's a lifeline for anyone walking through cancer, whether you're the patient or the person loving them through it. I wish every newly diagnosed person had this in their hands. Because of that, I'll be adding this to the resource page on the Test Those Breasts website so others navigating this journey can have access to it too.

—Jamie Vaughn
Breast Cancer Survivor
Founder & President, Test Those Breasts, Inc.

Dr. Troso has written an incredibly helpful guide for all of us facing a cancer diagnosis. Her compassion comes through just as strongly as her expertise on every page. I found myself referring to several chapters again and again as I progressed through my cancer journey, and gained so much clarity and knowledge as a result. I truly think this book would be an amazing gift and resource for anyone touched by cancer—patients, caregivers, and doctors alike!

—Becky Walker
Patient

Calming The Cancer Chaos

An Oncologist's Guide for Women to Understand, Organize, and Take Control of Their Cancer Care

TIFFANY TROSO-SANDOVAL, MD

Seshat Press
211 Pauline Drive #513
York, PA 17402
www.seshatpress.com
Send questions to: support@seshatpress.com

Paperback ISBN: 978-1-971288-08-6
eBook ISBN: 978-1-971288-09-3
Library of Congress Control Number: 2026919427

Seshat Press is proud to be a part of the Tree Neutral® program. Tree Neutral offsets the number of trees consumed in the production and printing of this book by taking proactive steps such as planting trees in direct proportion to the number of trees used to print books. To learn more about Tree Neutral, please visit treeneutral.com.

This book belongs to all of you. We wrote it together.

Contents

Preface

What I Want You to Know Before We Begin

Cancer is one of medicine's greatest challenges, but it is also one of medicine's greatest success stories. That success story is still being written, right now, for people like you. A cancer diagnosis does not mean today what it did a generation ago, or even a few years ago. The science has advanced, the treatments have changed, and survival outcomes have improved dramatically. Although cancer remains a serious illness, for the majority of people diagnosed today, it is treatable and frequently curable.

According to the American Cancer Society's most recent statistics report, the five-year relative survival rate for all cancers combined has now reached 70 percent, a dramatic improvement from just 49 percent in the mid-1970s (American Cancer Society 2026). That is not a small shift. That represents millions of people who are living full lives after a cancer diagnosis, people who were treated, who recovered, and who moved forward.

Advances in early detection, surgical techniques, targeted therapies, immunotherapy, and precision medicine have fundamentally changed what cancer looks like today (and we will discuss all of that). Some cancers that were once considered near-impossible to treat, such as certain types of lung cancer, liver cancer, and blood cancers like myeloma, have seen survival rates double or even triple in recent decades (American Cancer Society 2026). For many cancers, including breast and prostate, five-year survival rates now exceed 90 percent (Siegel et al. 2026).

It is equally important to understand that no two cancers are exactly alike. Lung cancer is not the same disease as breast cancer or uterine cancer, and even within a single cancer type, meaningful differences exist. Breast cancer, for example, includes multiple distinct subtypes, each with its own biology, behavior, and treatment approach. What works for one patient may not apply to another, even when the diagnosis appears similar on the surface.

This matters because your cancer journey is your own. Even if you find someone who shares your diagnosis, your stage, or even your specific subtype, your experience will still be uniquely yours. Your biology, your health history, your treatment response, and your path forward will differ in ways large and small. Comparing your journey to someone else's, whether in a waiting room or an online forum, rarely leads to clarity and often creates unnecessary fear or false expectations. The best guide to your situation is your own oncology team, working from your specific pathology, imaging, and health profile.

My goal is to help you understand your individual cancer diagnosis, organize your care, and engage meaningfully with the team that is guiding your treatment. Ultimately, I hope to help you obtain your best possible outcome while preserving your quality of life and remaining whole, not just as a patient, but as a person.

Introduction

The Appointment That Changed How I Practice Oncology

I'll never forget a woman I'll call Susan. She was fifty-two, newly diagnosed with Stage III ovarian cancer, and when she arrived for our first consultation, she was barely holding herself together. She'd spent three days on the internet, reading survival statistics and forums filled with worst-case scenarios. She was convinced she'd be dead within months and had already started writing goodbye letters to her teenage daughters.

I had nineteen patients scheduled that day. My nurse kept pointing at her watch. But something made me stop rushing.

I sat down across from Susan and asked, "What scares you most right now?"

She told me everything. The statistics she had read. Her aunt, who had died of ovarian cancer twenty years ago. The feeling that her body had betrayed her. The terror of leaving her daughters without a mother. The complete overwhelm of not knowing what came next.

So, I drew pictures. I explained what Stage III meant for her tumor type, not the aggregate data she'd found online. I walked through the treatment plan step by step: neoadjuvant chemo, surgery, more chemo. I drew a timeline on paper showing where we were starting and where we were headed. I explained that treatment had transformed dramatically since her aunt's death. I gave her a blank binder and planner, and we started filling them out together right there.

"I can't promise you a cure," I told her. "But I can promise you a plan, and I can promise you won't face this blindly. I am going to help you every step of the way, and I will answer all of your questions, as many times as you need, until you understand. And most of all, I promise that I will do everything that I can to help you get the best possible results from your treatments."

She stopped crying. She looked at the timeline and said, "No one explained it like this. I thought I was dying, and there was no hope. Now I actually feel like I have a plan and an expert as a partner."

That appointment ran over ninety minutes. I fell behind schedule, and my staff was frustrated. Nevertheless, afterwards, I had to retreat to my back office because my interaction with Susan was powerful and had taken a toll on me as well. I needed to regroup before I could resume seeing patients and continue to provide the same level of attentiveness and compassion.

Fortunately, Susan completed treatment and has been in remission for several years. But independent of her outcome, that appointment changed me. I realized that taking ninety minutes to truly educate one frightened patient wasn't inefficient. It was the most important thing I could do.

In addition to Susan, there were thousands more patients from whom I learned. Over twenty-five years of practicing medical oncology, specializing in breast and gynecological cancers at a major academic cancer institution, I've sat across the desk from countless women, each with her own fears, her own family, her own questions, her own way of facing the unimaginable. They gave me the privilege of being present in the most sacred moments of their lives, and every single one of them taught me something about what patients actually need from their oncologist. I learned which explanations worked and which created more confusion. They showed me what mattered most when facing mortality. I also learned that the manner in which I explained things, my tone, and my openness to listening to them all made a big difference.

This book exists because of them. Every organizational tool, every explanation, every piece of advice in these pages came from listening to thousands of patients who told me what helped, what didn't, what they wished they'd known sooner, and what made an impossible journey slightly more bearable.

The Emotions Are Real

Susan's story isn't unique. The emotions she felt that day (the terror, confusion, and overwhelming sense of being lost) are feelings I see in nearly every newly diagnosed patient who walks through my door. And they don't disappear just because treatment has started or even finished. If you're reading this book, you understand those feelings. Whether you're the one facing a cancer diagnosis or supporting someone who is, the emotions are real, powerful, and often frightening.

In my years of practice, I've worked with patients through every possible emotional reaction to cancer. What I've learned is that certain feelings appear almost universally, and recognizing them can be strangely comforting. You're not alone in what you're feeling. These are the emotions I see most often:

- **Terror that feels overwhelming.** Fear of the unknown. Fear of pain. Fear of what this means for your future and your family. This is the most common and immediate emotion.
- **Shock and disbelief.** "This can't be real. This can't be happening to me." Your mind struggles to accept information that fundamentally disrupts everything you thought you knew.
- **Anger at the unfairness.** "Why me? Why now?" You might feel angry at your body, angry at the universe, angry that this is happening when you have so much life left to live.
- **Complete overwhelm.** The sheer volume of medical terminology, appointments, and decisions feels like drinking from a fire hose. You know you need to act, but you don't know where to begin.
- **Loss of control.** Perhaps the most destabilizing feeling. Cancer didn't ask permission or consult your calendar. Suddenly, your life isn't entirely your own.
- **Profound isolation.** Even surrounded by loving family and friends, many patients describe feeling alone because no one else lives in your body or fully understands the private terror that wakes you at 3 a.m.
- **Guilt and self-blame.** "Did I cause this somehow?" This is almost never warranted, but it's incredibly common.

- **Confusion about the medical information.** Your doctor used terms you didn't understand, and you're left with more questions than answers.

If you're experiencing any or all of these emotions, you are having a completely normal reaction to an abnormal, life-altering situation. **The feelings themselves matter less than what we do with them. We can't always control our emotions, but we can control our response**. My goal is to empower you with hope, confidence, and clarity moving forward and to show you how to gather the information you need, how to build a team, make a plan, and move forward one step at a time.

What Calming the Cancer Chaos Actually Means

I chose this title carefully. I cannot eliminate the chaos of cancer: the unpredictability, the fear, the disruption to everything you thought your life would be. It will still be scary.

But I can give you tools to create pockets of order within that chaos:

- the planner that helps you track appointments and symptoms so you are not relying on memory during the brain fog of treatment
- the binder that organizes your records so you are not scrambling to find your pathology report at a consultation
- the knowledge that transforms medical jargon into something you can understand and discuss, and
- the questions that turn you from a passive recipient of care into an active participant in decisions about your body.

Calming the chaos means knowing what to expect at your first chemotherapy so it is slightly less terrifying. It means understanding what your staging means, so it is not just an abstract concept. It means having a plan, a timeline, and a team, so even when you are scared, you are not directionless. It means finding moments of clarity in the storm. And it means knowing that you have a map, even when the destination is uncertain.

Calming the Cancer Chaos is designed to guide you through your cancer journey chronologically, starting from the immediate aftermath of diagnosis through treatment, recovery, and surveillance. By walking you through each phase step by step, this book serves as both a roadmap and a reference, in language that is understandable.

I've also created a free companion workbook that is a practical and important component to help you get the most out of what you're about to learn. The workbook contains dozens of practical worksheets, templates, and organizational tools that transform the concepts in this book into systems you can easily use.

DOWNLOAD YOUR FREE COMPANION WORKBOOK HERE

Scan this QR code or go to www.calmingthecancerchaos.com/workbook

I hope you feel more prepared after reading these pages to ask questions and challenge assumptions when something does not make sense. I hope you feel equipped with practical tools to organize your care and communicate with your team. I hope you understand that being an informed patient does not mean becoming a medical expert, but knowing enough to participate meaningfully in your own decisions. And I hope you feel permission to have hard days, to ask for help, to say no to things that do not serve you, and to advocate fiercely for what you need.

Welcome to *Calming the Cancer Chaos.* You can do this. And I am going to help you.

Part I

Getting Oriented

Chapter 1

You're Not Alone: What to Expect from This Journey

You're Not Alone in This

If you're holding this book, something has happened that changed everything. Maybe you heard the words, "You have cancer," just days ago, and you're still moving through the world in a kind of fog, going through the motions while your mind keeps circling back to that moment in the doctor's office. Maybe you've known for a few weeks, and the initial shock is beginning to lift just enough to let the questions pour in. Or perhaps someone you love deeply is facing this diagnosis, and you're searching for ways to help.

Wherever you are right now, I want you to know: you are not lost, even if you feel that way. And you are not alone, even if it feels that way too.

There is a particular kind of fear that comes with a cancer diagnosis that is unlike almost anything else. It is not just fear of the disease itself. It is the fear of the unknown, the terror of sitting in a waiting room surrounded by people who all seem to know things you don't, the shame that creeps in when you didn't understand what your doctor just said but nodded anyway, the 3 a.m. moments when the house is quiet, and your mind is anything but. Every single one of those feelings makes complete sense. They are not signs of weakness.

They are completely valid, completely human responses to one of the hardest things a person can face.

What I have learned from my patients, over more than twenty-five years of sitting in the room with them, is that the fear does not disappear when you get more information. But it does change shape and becomes something you can work with, rather than something that is working against you. Even the smallest sense of a plan, even just knowing what the next step is, can shift you from feeling like the ground is gone from underneath you to feeling like you have somewhere to put your feet. That is what this book is for. Not to take away the hard parts, because I cannot promise that. But to make sure you never feel like a stranger in your own medical story.

I can promise you this: you are not behind. You do not need to have this figured out. You do not need to walk into your next appointment already knowing everything, already organized, already composed. You just need to take the next step, and I am going to walk through it with you.

What This Book Will Do for You

A cancer diagnosis does not come with a guidebook, although it should. What follows are the three things this book is designed to give you: clarity in a world that suddenly feels foreign, order in the middle of genuine chaos, and a way to show up in your own care as the informed, capable person you already are.

Goal 1: Transform Confusion Into Understanding

The vocabulary of oncology can feel like a foreign language at first. What does your pathology report actually mean? What is the difference between a surgical oncologist and a medical oncologist? Why are there so many different types of treatment, and how does your team decide which one is right for you? These are questions every patient deserves clear answers to, and as we work through them together, the conversations with your care team will feel less like trying to keep up and more like a genuine exchange. You will not become your own doctor. But you will understand enough to feel like yourself in the room.

Goal 2: Transform Chaos Into Organization

In the first weeks after a diagnosis, most women describe the same experience: a flood of appointments, phone calls, papers, and names they cannot keep straight. The medical system was not designed with your overwhelm in mind. It keeps moving whether you feel ready or not. The Cancer Journey Planner and the Cancer Journey Binder are the organizational tools woven throughout this book, and you will be prompted to update them often. Do the best that you can; it by no means has to be perfect. The purpose is to make it easy for you, so you always know where things are. Organization will not take away the hard parts of this journey, but it will help you maintain a sense of control, reduce anxiety, and create mental space to focus on what matters most.

Goal 3: Find Your Voice in This

There will be moments on this journey when you feel like things are simply happening to you, when the appointments blur together, the decisions feel too large, and the medical plan seems to be moving faster than you can follow. That feeling is real, and it makes complete sense. But your voice in this process matters more than you may realize right now. Your observations about your own body, your questions about your treatment, your instincts about what feels right—these are not interruptions to your care. They are part of it. Part of the book is about helping you find that voice and trust it: knowing when to ask, when to push, and when to lean on the expertise of the people around you. Empowerment means knowing what you can control, taking action in those areas, and letting go of what you can't control.

How This Book Is Organized

Calming the Cancer Chaos is structured to mirror your actual cancer journey, following the natural chronological progression from diagnosis through treatment to surveillance and beyond. This means that wherever you are right now, you can find the section that speaks directly to that moment.

The book is divided into four main parts:

- **Part I: Getting Oriented** helps you in the immediate aftermath of diagnosis, when everything feels uncertain, and the first question is simply: what do I do right now? You'll learn how to get organized, find the right doctors, and build your care team. This is the foundational work that sets you up for everything that follows.
- **Part II: Workup and Management** is for the diagnostic phase, when the tests, scans, and reports are coming in, and you are trying to make sense of what they mean. By the time you work through this section, the words on your medical reports will hopefully feel less like a foreign language and more like a map you know how to follow. This is where confusion transforms into clarity about your diagnosis and options.
- **Part III: Receiving Treatment** is intensely practical. When treatment begins, the questions shift from "What is happening?" to "How do I get through this?" These chapters stay close to the day-to-day reality of treatment: what to expect, how to manage side effects, and how to protect your energy for what matters most.
- **Part IV: Moving Forward-Reclaiming Your Health and Your Future** is for the phase that often catches people off guard. Finishing active treatment is not the same as the journey being over, and this section helps you navigate what comes next, from monitoring and surveillance to rebuilding your strength and finding your footing again.

By organizing this book in a chronological manner, I hope that it works both as a guide to read through and as a reference to return to whenever you need specific information. You do not have to read this book from beginning to end before it becomes useful. Start where you are. Turn to the section that meets you in this moment and let it walk with you from there.

Introducing Your Free Companion Workbook

Throughout this book, you will find references to a free companion workbook, available through the QR code at the end of this chapter or at **www.calmingthecancerchaos.com/workbook**. It contains the forms, checklists, and tracking templates that bring the organizational systems in these pages to life: medical history worksheets, symptom logs, appointment preparation guides, and more. The free workbook helps transform this book from a passive reading experience into an active, practical toolkit for managing your cancer care.

Think of this book as the *how-to* instruction manual, and the workbook as the actual tools you need to do the job.

Why the Workbook Matters So Much

Reading about organization is valuable, but actually having the organizational templates in your hands can be transformative. The workbook contains every form, worksheet, checklist, and template I reference throughout this book. Instead of staring at a blank piece of paper, wondering what to write, you simply fill in the blanks with forms designed by someone who's done this thousands of times.

This is important because, as you are going through cancer treatment, your time and energy are precious commodities. You don't have hours to spend creating tracking systems. The workbook does that work for you, saving you enormous amounts of time and mental energy that you can redirect toward healing.

But the real power of the workbook's contents is how they have the potential to facilitate and improve your medical care. How? Because good medicine depends on good information. When you arrive with a completed medical history worksheet, your oncologist immediately has a clear picture. When you track symptoms in the provided log, your doctor can see patterns that help them adjust medications or catch problems early. When you bring organized questions, nothing important gets overlooked.

Just as importantly, the workbook reduces anxiety. Anxiety thrives on uncertainty and disorganization. When you're trying to hold dozens of details in your head, your brain constantly worries you'll forget something critical. When you write things down in organized systems, you externalize that information, and your brain no longer has to hold it all. The peace of mind that comes from knowing you are organized and that nothing is slipping through the cracks is invaluable.

Good medical care is a partnership, and the pages in the workbook give you the tools to advocate effectively for yourself.

What's Actually in the Workbook

The companion workbook contains dozens of printable worksheets, forms, and templates designed to support you at every phase of your journey, including:

- tools to get you organized from day one, like comprehensive medical history forms, medication tracking sheets, and contact lists for your healthcare team,
- preparation guides for medical appointments, so you show up ready with the right questions, the right documents, and the confidence that you won't forget anything important,
- daily and weekly tracking logs to monitor your symptoms, treatment cycles, side effects, and overall patterns, so your medical team has the detailed information they need to help you,
- organizational systems, including binder setup guides, financial trackers, and calendars specifically designed for managing cancer treatment schedules,
- long-term planning resources for post-treatment surveillance, advance care planning, and reflection tools to help you process the emotional aspects of your journey.

Each tool can be printed as many times as you need and customized to fit your specific situation. Use what serves you; skip what doesn't.

At the end of this chapter, you'll find another QR code. Using your smartphone camera, simply point it at the code, and it will automatically open a link to the workbook download page.

Once you click the link, you'll download the complete workbook as a PDF file. If possible, then transfer it to your computer or tablet for easy viewing. Otherwise, you can also download it directly from the following website page: https://www.calmingthecancerchaos.com/workbook

Next, you can:

- print the entire workbook and keep it in a three-ring binder
- print individual worksheets as needed
- fill out some forms digitally before printing
- share relevant pages with family members, helping you stay organized.

How to Best Use This Book

The most effective way to use this book depends on where you are in your cancer journey.

If You've Just Been Diagnosed

Start with Part I to get organized and build your care team. Download the workbook and complete the foundational forms (Medical History, Medication List, Healthcare Provider Contacts) before your first oncology appointments. Then read ahead to the chapters that address what's coming next in your specific treatment plan.

If You're Already in Treatment

Jump directly to the section that addresses where you are now. If you're receiving chemotherapy, go to Part III. If you're between diagnosis and treatment, start with Part II. Then circle back to set up the organizational systems in Part I. It's never too late to get organized, and you'll immediately feel the benefit.

If You're Supporting a Loved One

Read the book through from beginning to end to understand the full journey your loved one is facing. Download the workbook and offer to help set up and maintain the organizational systems. Many patients feel too overwhelmed to do this alone, and having a helper makes an enormous difference. Focus especially on the preparation checklists so you can help them get ready for appointments.

The Book as an Ongoing Reference

Please do not feel you need to read this book cover to cover before it becomes useful. It's designed to be a resource you return to repeatedly. Keep it accessible. When questions arise, when you need to prepare for a specific appointment, or when you're facing a new phase of treatment, turn to the relevant section. The chronological structure makes it easy to find what you need when you need it.

What This Book Can Do and What It Cannot Do

This book can help you understand your diagnosis in clear terms, organize your medical information, prepare for each phase of treatment, advocate for yourself effectively, manage side effects, and reduce anxiety through knowledge and preparation.

This book cannot replace your oncology team's medical advice, tell you which treatment to choose, guarantee any particular outcome, address every possible cancer scenario, eliminate all fear, or answer every specific question about your unique situation. Those questions need to be asked of your oncology team, who know your specific case.

Think of this book as a knowledgeable guide walking beside you, explaining the terrain and pointing out what to watch for. But your oncology team provides your actual medical care. This book supports that partnership. It doesn't replace it.

Moving Forward

The fact that you're here, reading this book, tells me something important about you. You're someone who wants to understand, who wants to be prepared, and who wants to face this challenge as an informed participant rather than a passive patient. That mindset is one of your greatest assets.

Over the next few chapters, we're going to build on that foundation. You'll learn the vocabulary of cancer care, discover practical tools for staying organized, understand what each member of your care team does, and prepare for treatment. Most importantly, you'll develop confidence that even though you didn't choose this journey, you can navigate it with knowledge, support, and a clear plan.

Your First Action Item: The Baseline Self-Assessment

In your companion workbook, you'll find a single-page tool called the **Baseline Self-Assessment Checklist**. This simple worksheet asks you to name where you are in your journey and rate the emotions you may be carrying with you: rate everything from shock, anger, and overwhelm to hope and determination.

This takes less than five minutes, but it will be very helpful going forward. Make sure to answer it honestly. There are no right or wrong answers, just how you truly feel and think.

Cancer treatment can be a long road, and in the middle of it, sometimes you may feel like you are not making progress. You'll have hard days when the fear feels just as intense as it did at the beginning. In those moments, I want you to pull out this assessment and look at what you wrote today. You'll see how far you've really come. The confusion that feels overwhelming right now will have transformed into understanding. The fear will have shifted into something more manageable. Your own handwriting will prove your resilience.

WORKBOOK CHECKPOINT: Please find your **Baseline Self-Assessment Checklist** on workbook page 1/1.

Many of my patients tell me that revisiting this assessment months later becomes one of the most powerful moments of their journey. They can barely remember feeling as lost as they did on day one. But seeing it written down reminds them of how much they've grown, how much they've learned, and how much stronger they've become.

You didn't choose this path. But you are choosing how to walk it. Let's walk it together, informed, organized, and prepared for whatever comes next. There is a lot to be hopeful for, and I am rooting for you. Let's get started.

DOWNLOAD YOUR FREE COMPANION WORKBOOK HERE

Scan this QR code or go to www.calmingthecancerchaos.com/workbook

Chapter 2

Creating Order from Chaos: Your Organizational System

As you navigate the challenging path of cancer treatment, the importance of maintaining control over numerous details and decisions cannot be overstated. Organization can be an important tool in your journey, offering a way to bring order to the chaos and empowering you to manage the complexities of your care with more confidence and clarity. In this chapter, I will review my two favorite tools for patients: **The Cancer Journey Planner** and **The Cancer Journey Binder,** which can be found in the workbook Chapter 2 on pages 1, 2 and 3.

The Cancer Journey Planner

The planner is a structured approach to creating a much-needed foundation of stability, allowing you to focus on healing while still participating in the aspects of life that bring you joy and fulfillment. By writing down your appointments on a schedule and documenting your side effects in real time, there is much less information that you need to maintain in your short-term memory. This will free up space in your mind to allow room for other, more enjoyable things, as well as reduce your worry. By writing it all down in the planner, you will alleviate some stress and anxiety.

Here are some examples of how a well-organized and clearly scheduled approach can significantly benefit various facets of your cancer journey. More detailed explanations of how to implement them will follow.

- **Chemotherapy Treatment Schedules**: Keeping a detailed schedule of your chemotherapy treatments, including dates, times, and any pre- or post-treatment medications, is crucial. This helps increase the likelihood that your treatment will proceed as planned, minimizing the risk of complications and enhancing its effectiveness. It also facilitates clear communication with your healthcare team about your treatment progress and any concerns that may arise.
- **Managing Conflicting Appointments**: With visits to various specialists, tests, and treatments, an organized calendar is vital. It helps you prevent overlapping appointments, ensuring that each aspect of your care receives the attention it deserves without the added stress of last-minute rescheduling.
- **Tracking Symptoms and Side Effects**: A daily log of how you feel and any treatment reactions you experience is invaluable for your care team. This information can highlight patterns and help adjust your treatment plan, making your journey more manageable.
- **Making Time for Family, Holidays, and Work**: Perhaps most important, an organized approach allows you to carve out precious time for significant life events. This could be a family gathering, a holiday celebration, or necessary work commitments. Having a clear overview of your schedule allows you to plan these moments, ensuring that cancer doesn't rob you of the joys and responsibilities of everyday life.

In summary, organization is more than a logistical necessity; it is your strategy to maintain engagement with the life you cherish. By keeping a tight schedule and a clear record, you not only optimize your care but also preserve space for the moments that feed your spirit and sustain your resolve to fight.

For this purpose, I recommend purchasing a weekly/monthly planner. These are readily available at online vendors, a local office supply store, or from my online store (the link is in your workbook with the corresponding pages for this chapter).

How to Use Your Cancer Journey Planner

Monthly Pages

- Document **all** appointments related to cancer treatment.
- Highlight treatment days in yellow.
- Highlight important holidays, birthdays, and family events in another color.

> **PRO TIP:** For chemotherapy treatment dates, list the cycle number so you can keep track.

Weekly Pages

- Mark each day with the cycle day (how many days since your last treatment). For example, if you had chemotherapy on Monday, March 11 (day zero), then Tuesday, March 12, is day one. Document any prominent symptoms, for example:
    - **Nausea**: How often, how severe, did antinausea medicine work?
    - **Bowel movements**: Hard stool, loose stool? If diarrhea, how many times? Did you take anything for either symptom, and did it work?
    - **Neuropathy**: Numbness or tingling, or pain in fingers and toes.
    - **Bone pain**: Severity, location. Did you take anything?
    - **Fatigue**: Grade it on a scale from one to five, with five being unable to get out of bed.

    - **Mouth sores**: How many, where (tongue, gums, or roof of mouth), what did they look like?
- Document any other important things to track for yourself. (*Check with your doctor*). For example, if you have diabetes, then maybe list your blood sugar levels once or twice a day, or if you have high blood pressure, write it down.
- Document hydration. I recommend that you keep track of how much water you drink. Most patients should aim for at least **two liters** (approximately sixty-seven ounces per day). *But please check with your own doctor about how much water to drink,* especially in the setting of other complicating factors, such as kidney or heart disease.
- Bring the planner with you to each visit to share with your healthcare provider. As a physician, it is much easier to help you with a symptom if it's tracked and quantified as above. This provides us with specific information about your symptom, so that we can best help you. For example, a patient who has a lot of nausea the day after treatment would possibly be given a different treatment than someone who develops nausea on day four.

Now that you understand how powerful a well-organized planner can be, let's make sure you set yours up correctly from day one.

In your companion workbook, you'll find the **Cancer Journey Planner Setup Guide**—a step-by-step visual checklist that walks you through purchasing the right planner, setting up your color-coding system, and creating sample monthly and weekly page layouts. You'll also find the **Daily Symptom and Wellness Tracker**, a printable log page you can use right now if you haven't purchased a planner yet, or as a detailed supplement to your planner pages.

These two tools transform the concept of *tracking symptoms* into a concrete, manageable system. Instead of staring at blank planner pages, wondering what to write, you'll have clear examples and structured templates that make tracking effortless.

Consider completing the Planner Setup Guide before your next appointment. Many patients tell me that setting up their planner reduced their anxiety more than almost anything else because it gave them a sense of control over the chaos, as well as a better tool for communication with their physician.

The Cancer Journey Binder

What nobody tells you at the beginning is that your doctors do not automatically talk to each other, and not all hospitals work on the same system. Imaging done at one facility may not be visible to a specialist at another. A medication prescribed by your surgeon may not appear in your oncologist's notes. Test results get faxed, lost, or filed somewhere no one thinks to look. This is not anyone's fault. It is simply how a complex medical system works, and it means that without someone actively keeping track of the full picture, important information can slip through the cracks.

This brings me to the second part of your organizational plan, which is **The Cancer Journey Binder**. In today's rapidly evolving healthcare landscape, I feel it is important for you to maintain an organized collection of your own medical records. When the important parts of your medical chart travel with you, you walk into every appointment as the most informed person in the room. Your doctors spend less time hunting for information and more time focused on your care.

In my experience, there are three specific ways a well-maintained binder makes a direct difference in the quality of your care:

- **Enhancing Accuracy During Medical Consultations**: By having immediate access to your medical history, you enhance the accuracy of your consultations. It's not uncommon to see multiple specialists, and details can be overlooked or forgotten. As a physician, I have found that even with electronic medical records, it can be difficult to dig out the most important and necessary documents among hundreds of pages of scanned files. By maintaining a comprehensive record, you ensure that each healthcare provider is fully informed about your medical history, current medications, allergies, and past procedures.

- **Improving Emergency Preparedness**: In emergency situations, time is of the essence. Having organized medical records readily available can be lifesaving. For example, if you're unconscious or unable to communicate, emergency medical personnel can quickly access your medical history, chronic conditions, allergies, or medications that might influence treatment options. Such preparation can significantly impact outcomes in critical situations.
- **Empowering You to Advocate for Yourself**: Maintaining personal medical records helps you remain engaged and become your own best advocate. It enables you to track your treatment progress, understand your condition better, and ask specific, informed questions during medical appointments. Your active involvement can help you be better equipped to express your concerns, preferences, and observations. Basically, by following these guidelines, you are helping your doctor to best help you. It also fosters a sense of control over your health journey, which can be particularly empowering during cancer treatment when so much feels out of your control.

Here is a brief guide to creating and assembling your **Cancer Journey Binder,** with step-by-step instructions below and in the workbook:

1. Begin with a sturdy two-inch wide, three-ring binder for a physical space to hold your journey's narrative. You will also need a three-hole punch for your documents' new home, with tabbed dividers to categorize your medical story, and a label maker or Sharpie for clear, lasting labels. A highlighter will call attention to crucial information (such as report dates and type of report) for filing purposes, and

binder folders with zip closures to safeguard small, irregular items that need to be kept and easily accessible.

2. Your binder should have several sections, each marked by a tabbed divider labeled with important aspects of your care: doctors, meds/allergies, pathology, genetics, radiology, Dr. notes, treatment plan/drugs, and labs. These sections will organize your documents, making each piece of information readily accessible whenever you need it.
3. As you gather documents, sort them by the type of information they contain, matching the labels on your dividers. In each section, arrange the documents chronologically, with the most recent on top, so your medical history unfolds in reverse chronological order, keeping your most current information at your fingertips.
4. Insert your sorted documents into the binder, using the three-hole punch to secure them in place. For items that don't fit the standard mold—like CDs from radiological exams, or small notes, or business cards—use the binder pockets.

PRO TIP: Whenever you undergo a radiological exam, request a copy of the exam on a disk right when you check in. Make sure to collect the disk before you leave the facility. This small act ensures you have a complete visual history of your scans, which can be invaluable for consultations or future treatments.

I truly believe that your **Cancer Journey Binder** is more than just a collection of documents; it's your tool for empowerment, a record of your resilience, and a testament to your proactive role in your healthcare journey.

How to Create and Use Your Cancer Journey Binder

1. Purchase binder and supplies:
   - Two-inch wide, three-ring binder
   - Three-hole punch
   - Tabbed dividers
   - Label maker or Sharpie
   - Highlighter
   - Plastic binder folders with zip closure
2. Label divider tabs as follows:
   - Doctors
   - Meds/Allergies
   - Pathology
   - Genetics
   - Radiology
   - Notes
   - Treatment Plan/Drugs
   - Labs
3. Sort your documents according to:
   - Type of document based on labels above
   - Sort each group by date, with the most recent on top
4. Insert documents into binder:
   - Three-hole punch pages evenly by first stacking them neatly together so the holes all line up once punched
   - Use binder pockets to hold irregular-sized items that are important to keep, such as disks from radiological exams

Examples of Document Types for Sorting

- **Doctors:** List name, office info, phone, fax, and type of doctor/ specialty for each doctor you have seen in the last two years. Better to include more than less.

- **Meds/Allergies:** List **all** medications that you take, including doses and how often taken. Consider also including what it is used for and when you started taking it. Also, list **all** supplements and vitamins, **and** anything you take just when you need it, such as Advil, Pepcid, etc. Aim for completeness.
- List any medication allergies and what the allergic reaction entails, i.e., swelling, rash, shortness of breath, etc.
- **Pathology:** Pathological report, Cytology, FNA (fine needle aspiration), Core biopsy
- **Genetics:** Myriad, foundation, Cyrus, DNA molecular profile report, genomic report, next-generation sequencing
- **Radiology:** CT scan, PET scan, MRI, ultrasound, X-rays, mammogram
- **Doctor's notes:** These may be trickier to obtain, but always ask the office secretary for a copy of any initial consultation and ask intermittently (every six to twelve weeks) for a copy from the most recent office visit. Sometimes these are also downloadable from an online chart. Also request any operative notes from major surgeries and procedure notes, such as from a paracentesis/thoracentesis (drainage of fluid), placement of a mediport or catheter.
- **Treatment Plan/Drugs:** Chemotherapy and/or treatment records, drug information on medications you will be receiving (ondansetron, tamoxifen, Adriamycin). Also include any instructions on how to manage expected side effects.
- **Labs:** intermittent CBC (complete blood count), Chemistry/Comprehensive panel (do **not** save every lab report).
- Save the first set and then every six to twelve weeks. Tumor markers are often monitored and should be saved each time they are drawn. Examples include: CA125, CEA, CA15-3, CA27-29, CA19-9. Doctors don't draw these at every visit, and what is drawn will be different depending on the type of cancer for which the patient is being treated.

Taking Action: Build Your Organizational Foundation Today

You now understand why I believe the Cancer Journey Planner and Cancer Journey Binder are important tools and how they work together to bring order to chaos, reduce anxiety, and potentially even improve your medical care. But understanding alone won't help you. You also need to create these systems.

WORKBOOK CHECKPOINT: Hopefully, the instructions above are clear, but to make it more actionable, you can find three tools for Chapter 2 in your workbook:

- Page 2/1, **Cancer Journey Planner Setup Guide:** A visual, step-by-step checklist with sample monthly and weekly page layouts, color-coding instructions, and symptom tracking guidelines. This tool shows you exactly how to set up your planner so it works for you from day one.
- Page 2/2, **Daily Symptom and Wellness Tracker:** A printable daily log page you can start using immediately (even before you get a planner). Make multiple copies and complete one each day during treatment. This becomes your goldmine of data for your medical team.
- Page 2/3, **Cancer Journey Binder Assembly Checklist and Document Sorting Guide:** A comprehensive guide that includes a shopping list, tab setup instructions, document-by-document filing guidance, and a visual diagram of what a completed binder looks like. This eliminates all the guesswork.

DOWNLOAD YOUR FREE COMPANION WORKBOOK HERE

Scan this QR code or go to www.calmingthecancerchaos.com/workbook

Chapter 3

Finding Your Partners in This Fight: Building a Team You Can Trust

In the first days after a diagnosis, before treatment has even begun, you are already being asked to make decisions that feel impossibly large. Which doctor do you go to? Do you stay close to home or travel to a major cancer center? Does it matter? Should you get a second opinion, and if so, will that offend your doctor? These choices may shape not only your treatment options but also your experience along the way. The right team combines medical expertise with a personal style that matches your needs and values.

In this chapter, we will walk through who the different specialists are and what each of them actually does, some of the differences are between a private practice and an academic cancer center, and how to walk into your first consultation feeling prepared rather than caught off guard. By the time you finish, my goal is for you to have a clear sense of what to look for, what to ask, and how to build a team that you genuinely trust.

The Oncology Specialists You'll Meet

Cancer care involves a team of doctors, each with a specific role. Understanding who they are and what they do helps you feel more in control of the process.

- **Surgical Oncologists** are the surgeons who focus on cancer. They are the ones you see when surgery is part of your treatment. Sometimes their role is to remove the entire tumor, and other times it may be to perform a biopsy that helps confirm your diagnosis.
- **Medical Oncologists** specialize in treating cancer with medications such as chemotherapy, hormone therapy, immunotherapy, and targeted therapies. They are often your main oncologist, responsible for coordinating your overall treatment plan. You can think of the medical oncologist as the conductor of your care, making sure the different parts of treatment work together.
- **Radiation Oncologists** use high-energy radiation to target and destroy cancer cells. Radiation may be given alone or combined with surgery or medications. These specialists carefully design your treatment so that the radiation is aimed precisely at the tumor while limiting exposure to normal tissue.

Most often, your treatment plan is created by a **multidisciplinary team**. Surgical, medical, and radiation oncologists work together to decide the best sequence and combination of treatments. Each specialist brings their own expertise, and together they create a plan tailored to you.

Choosing Your Treatment Arena: Private Practice Versus Academic Centers

The setting in which you receive your care, whether a private practice or an academic center, can significantly influence your treatment experience. In many cases, you may not have the luxury of choice between different treatment settings due to availability in your area, especially in rural communities. What matters most is that you feel comfortable with your doctor, reassured about their expertise in your specific type of cancer, and confident in their ability to explain your care.

Private practices often stand out for their personalized approach. A smaller-scale facility can translate to more direct interaction with your oncologist and an intimate care environment. Flexibility and ease of scheduling may also be added perks. However, private practices might not always have immediate access to the latest therapies or clinical trials and may not be equipped for the most complex cases. This is a vast generalization, and I certainly cannot speak for all private practices, so ultimately, you will need to evaluate the private practices in your area.

Academic centers, often affiliated with universities, are the powerhouses of cancer research and innovation. These institutions offer access not only to current treatments but also to the next generation of therapies through clinical trials. They can be particularly beneficial for those with rare cancers or complex cases. The trade-off is that the environment may feel more impersonal, and with multiple oncologists, physician assistants, nurse practitioners, and fellows involved, you might not always see the same doctor.

If your situation is complex, or if you are interested in clinical trials, an academic center may be advantageous. Regardless, I always recommend that you seek a second opinion, particularly from an academic center, since this provides a broader perspective about your treatment options and adds confidence in the path you are following.

To see how these differences between private practices and academic centers play out in real life, let's look at two women who faced similar choices but made different decisions.

Patient Spotlight: Maria's Choice of a Private Practice

Maria, a fifty-two-year-old teacher, was diagnosed with early-stage breast cancer. She chose to be treated at a private oncology practice close to home. What mattered most to her was personal attention and being able to reach her doctor quickly with questions. The convenience of not traveling into the city and the strong relationship she built with her oncologist gave her the reassurance she needed. For her stage and type of cancer, standard therapies were very effective, so she didn't feel she was missing out by not being at a large academic center.

Patient Spotlight: Elaine's Path to an Academic Center

Elaine, aged forty-seven, learned she had a rare type of ovarian cancer. Her doctor at a private practice recommended that she seek a second opinion at a nearby academic center, since they might have access to clinical trials not available in smaller settings. At the academic center, Elaine was offered the chance to join a study testing a new drug designed specifically for her cancer type. She decided to transfer her care there to access the trial. Importantly, her private practice doctor supported this decision and remained part of her broader care circle. Elaine learned that seeking a second opinion is not about dissatisfaction with your doctor; rather, it is about making sure you have every option available to you.

Maximizing Your Consultations

To forge a productive partnership with your oncologist, preparation is key. Here's how you can get ready:

First: Be Prepared to Tell Your Oncologist All About You!

Your Medical History: A Comprehensive Story

Your oncologist needs to see your full health history to tailor your treatment accurately. This includes chronic conditions, previous illnesses, past surgeries, and any other relevant medical events. A detailed health chronicle helps your oncologist understand your cancer and you as a whole person, ensuring a safe, calculated approach to your treatment.

WORKBOOK CHECKPOINT: In your companion workbook on page 3/1, you will find the **Complete Medical History Worksheet**, a comprehensive form designed specifically for cancer patients that captures almost everything your oncologist needs to know. Patients who arrive with this completed often have better first appointment experiences because more time can be spent discussing diagnosis and treatment instead of spending precious appointment time gathering basic information. If possible, try to complete this worksheet before your first appointment. It takes twenty to thirty minutes and will be valuable for you going forward.

Medications and Allergies

Your medication list matters more than most patients expect. Every prescription, every over-the-counter remedy, every vitamin and supplement needs to be on that list, along with the dose and how often you take it. Your oncologist is looking for interactions, contraindications, and gaps in your care that may not be obvious to anyone except the person who can see everything at once. That person, right now, is you.

Allergies belong on that list too, with as much detail as you can remember: the name of the medication, what happened, and when. This level of detail matters because not all reactions carry the same weight. A childhood reaction to penicillin and a recent severe reaction to carboplatin chemotherapy are very different pieces of information with very different implications for your treatment. When in doubt, write it down and let your oncologist sort out what is relevant.

One more thing worth doing before your first appointment is pulling together your vaccine history. It may not feel connected to your cancer care, but treatment can affect how your immune system responds to infection, and your oncologist will want to know where you stand before making decisions about your care. This information can usually be obtained from your primary care provider or even from the local pharmacy where you may have received the vaccines.

WORKBOOK CHECKPOINT: Medication and Allergy Worksheet is on page 3/2.

WORKBOOK CHECKPOINT: The My Vaccine History is on page 3/3.

Other Healthcare Providers: Building a Coordinated Team

An often overlooked yet essential part of your medical documentation is a list of other healthcare providers involved in your care. This includes specialists (i.e., cardiologist, pulmonologist, endocrinologist, neurologist), general practitioners, and any other medical professionals **you see regularly**. Providing your oncologist with this information facilitates seamless communication between the members of your healthcare team. It ensures that everyone is on the same page regarding your treatment to avoid potential overlaps or conflicts in your care plan.

WORKBOOK CHECKPOINT: A Healthcare Provider Contact Form is available on page 3/5.

Patient Spotlight: Lydia

When Lydia, age forty-five, first noticed a lump in her breast, she was terrified. Her biopsy revealed triple-negative breast cancer, and further testing showed it had already spread to a lymph node. Because of the size and aggressiveness of her tumor, her doctors recommended chemotherapy and immunotherapy before surgery.

Lydia came to her first consultation with a detailed health history, a written list of her medications and supplements, and questions about her family history of cancer. She had also asked her oncologist's office ahead of time what records they would need and brought them organized in a binder. This preparation mattered. Her oncologist immediately recommended genetic testing, which revealed a PALB2 gene mutation, which affects how a cell repairs its DNA. This information shaped both her surgery and her long-term risk management.

Over the next year, Lydia's journey included chemotherapy, a bilateral mastectomy, radiation, and maintenance immunotherapy. Because she had asked about coordination of care early on, she was also referred to a gynecologic oncologist to discuss preventive removal of her ovaries and tubes. She also asked about seeing a nutritionist, a social worker, and for a referral to integrative medicine! Lydia's preparation at her first few visits gave her team a clear picture of her health, allowed them to anticipate her needs, and helped her feel like a true partner in her treatment.

Second: Have Your Questions Ready!

Asking the Right Questions

Consultations often move quickly, and it's easy to leave with some confusion and unanswered questions. Having a clear set of questions ensures that you not only understand your diagnosis but also what lies ahead in terms of treatment, side effects, and long-term planning. In addition, think about what you need to know, not only from a medical perspective but also in terms of how treatment will affect your daily life. Here I list some of the most important things to cover in your consultation. I also have a downloadable resource in the workbook.

Understanding Your Diagnosis

Begin by asking your doctor to explain your pathology report in clear terms. Confirm the exact type and stage of cancer, and what additional tests may be necessary to complete your workup. In some cases, you may want to ask whether genetic testing is appropriate for you or whether your tumor will be analyzed for DNA mutations that could influence treatment.

Exploring Treatment Options

Once you understand your diagnosis, ask about the standard treatment plan for your specific type and stage of cancer. Find out whether clinical trials are available and if they might be appropriate for you. Some patients also want to know whether a repeat biopsy is recommended before starting therapy.

Clarifying Treatment Details

You'll want to understand the logistics of your care. How many treatments will you need? How often will they take place, and where will they be given? Will any part of your treatment require hospitalization? These details help you prepare practically and emotionally.

Anticipating Side Effects

Every treatment has potential side effects, both short-term and long-term. Ask your oncologist to provide written instructions on how to manage them. Find out how treatment may affect your daily life, work, travel, or even holding your child. The more you know upfront, the better prepared you'll feel.

Looking Ahead at Outcomes

It's reasonable to ask about expected outcomes. What is your prognosis with the recommended treatment? How will your team measure whether it is working? How often will scans or bloodwork be performed, and will your oncologist use newer tools such as ctDNA (circulating tumor DNA) for monitoring?

Managing Practical Concerns

Cancer care often comes with financial questions. Clarify whether your insurance covers the proposed treatments and whether there are additional costs to anticipate. If necessary, you should ask if the practice has a financial counselor, navigator, or social worker who can help you explore these issues.

Integrating Treatment Into Your Life

Your health extends beyond cancer. Ask whether you should adjust your diet, whether it is safe to continue exercising, and how treatment may affect your ability to work or travel. Many centers have nutritionists, counselors, or support groups that can help you adjust.

Understanding Your Care Team

Finally, ask about the people who will be involved in your care. Who will you see regularly, and how can you best communicate with them? Will your oncologist be present at every step, or will nurse practitioners and physician assistants play a large role? Clarify how to reach your team outside of office hours and which hospitals your doctor is affiliated with.

WORKBOOK CHECKPOINT: First Consultation Preparation and Essential Questions is on page 3/4 in your workbook.

Special Considerations for Younger Women: Fertility Preservation

If you are of childbearing age and considering future pregnancies, then one of the first conversations you should have with your oncologist is about fertility preservation. Cancer treatment can damage the ovaries and reduce or eliminate your ability to conceive in the future. For some women, treatment may bring on early menopause. The emotional weight of potentially losing fertility on top of a cancer diagnosis can feel overwhelming, but knowing your options and acting quickly can preserve future possibilities.

The critical point is that fertility preservation must happen before you start treatment. Once chemotherapy begins, the window closes. That's why this conversation needs to happen early (ideally at your first or second oncology appointment), even if you're not sure whether you want children or more children in the future. Circumstances and feelings can change, and protecting the option to choose later is empowering.

Why Cancer Treatment Affects Fertility

Chemotherapy drugs are designed to target rapidly dividing cells, which include cancer cells but also the eggs in your ovaries. Unlike men, who produce new sperm continuously throughout life, women are born with all the eggs they will ever have. Chemotherapy can damage or destroy these eggs, and depending on the drugs used, the dosage, and your age, the impact can range from temporary fertility disruption to permanent infertility.

Hormone therapy, particularly treatments that suppress ovarian function or block estrogen, can also affect fertility. Even radiation therapy, if directed at the pelvis, can damage the ovaries or uterus. The younger you are, the more eggs you typically have in reserve, but there are no guarantees.

Options for Preserving Fertility

Several options exist, and the best choice depends on your diagnosis, treatment timeline, relationship status, personal preferences, and financial considerations. A reproductive endocrinologist who specializes in fertility will guide you through the process and work with your oncologist to coordinate timing.

Egg Freezing (Oocyte Cryopreservation)

This is the most common option for women without a partner or who prefer not to use donor sperm. The process involves stimulating your ovaries with hormone injections for about ten to fourteen days, monitoring your response with ultrasounds and blood tests, and then retrieving the mature eggs through a minor outpatient procedure. The eggs are frozen and stored for future use. When you're ready to use them, they can be thawed, fertilized with sperm, and transferred to your uterus as embryos.

The advantage of egg freezing is that it preserves your genetic material without requiring a partner. The challenge is that it requires a window of time before treatment starts, and not all treatment plans can be delayed. Additionally, success rates depend on the number and quality of eggs retrieved, which varies by age.

Embryo Freezing (Embryo Cryopreservation)

For women who have a partner or are comfortable using donor sperm, embryo freezing may be an option. The process is similar to egg freezing, but the eggs are fertilized with sperm in the lab before being frozen. Some patients prefer this because embryos tend to survive the freezing and thawing process slightly better than unfertilized eggs, though modern techniques have narrowed that gap significantly.

Embryo freezing also requires the same ten- to fourteen-day timeline, and you'll need to make decisions about what happens to the embryos if your circumstances change (for example, if a relationship ends).

Ovarian Tissue Cryopreservation

This is a newer and less commonly used option, but it can be valuable for women who cannot delay treatment long enough for egg or embryo freezing. In this procedure, a piece of your ovary is surgically removed, frozen, and stored. Later, after cancer treatment is complete, the tissue can be thawed and transplanted back into the body, where it may restore hormone production and, in some cases, allow for natural conception.

This option is still considered experimental in many centers, and success rates vary. However, it's an important choice for prepubescent girls, women facing immediate chemotherapy, or those with certain types of cancer where hormone stimulation (required for egg freezing) is not safe.

Ovarian Suppression During Chemotherapy

Some oncologists may offer medications called GnRH agonists (such as leuprolide or goserelin) to temporarily *shut down* the ovaries during chemotherapy. The theory is that putting the ovaries into a temporary menopausal state may protect them from chemotherapy damage. However, the evidence supporting this approach is mixed, and it should not be considered a reliable method of fertility preservation. If you are interested in preserving fertility, eggs, or embryos, then freezing remains the gold standard.

Timing and Coordination

The biggest challenge with fertility preservation is time. Some women feel pressured to start cancer treatment immediately and worry that delaying even two weeks is dangerous. In most cases, a brief delay of ten to fourteen days for egg or embryo freezing will not significantly impact your cancer outcomes, especially in early-stage disease. Your oncologist and fertility specialist will work together to determine whether this window is safe for you.

If your cancer is more advanced or aggressive, ovarian tissue cryopreservation may be the only option, since it can be done quickly and doesn't require hormonal stimulation. In rare cases, fertility preservation may not be possible, and your oncologist will be honest with you about those limitations.

Financial and Insurance Considerations

Fertility preservation can be expensive, with costs ranging from several thousand to over ten thousand dollars, depending on the procedure and how many cycles are needed. Some insurance plans cover fertility preservation for cancer patients, but many do not. Several nonprofit organizations offer grants and financial assistance programs specifically for cancer patients pursuing fertility preservation. Your fertility clinic's financial counselor can help you explore these options.

Some states have laws requiring insurance companies to cover fertility preservation for medical reasons, including cancer treatment. Ask your oncology team's social worker or patient navigator to help you understand what is available in your state.

The Emotional Complexity of the Decision

Deciding whether to pursue fertility preservation can feel overwhelming. You may not know if you want children in the future, or you may feel conflicted about focusing on fertility when you're trying to process a cancer diagnosis. Some women feel guilty for *thinking about tomorrow* when they're not even sure about today.

It's important to give yourself permission to consider all your options without judgment. Fertility preservation is not about making a final decision on parenthood right now; rather, it is about keeping that door open. Even if you ultimately decide not to use the preserved eggs or embryos, many women find comfort in knowing they had the choice.

If you are struggling with this decision, consider speaking with a counselor, a trusted friend, or other cancer survivors who faced similar choices. Your oncology team can also connect you with support resources.

Questions to Ask Your Oncologist and Fertility Specialist

- Will my cancer treatment affect my fertility? If so, how likely is it?
- Is there time to pursue fertility preservation before starting treatment?
- Can you refer me to a reproductive endocrinologist who works with cancer patients?
- What fertility preservation options are best for my situation?
- How long will the process take, and will it delay my cancer treatment?
- Are there risks to fertility preservation given my type of cancer?
- Does my insurance cover fertility preservation for medical reasons?
- What financial assistance programs are available?
- If I cannot pursue fertility preservation now, are there other options later?

Moving Forward

Fertility preservation is a deeply personal decision, and there is no right or wrong answer. What matters is that you have the information, the time to consider your options, and the support to make the choice that feels right for you. If preserving fertility is important to you, bring it up at your very first appointment. Don't wait for your doctor to mention it. You must advocate for yourself and ask the questions that matter most to your future.

In Summary

Choosing the right doctors and treatment setting is one of the most important decisions you will make in your cancer journey. Understanding the roles of surgical, medical, and radiation oncologists allows you to see how each specialist contributes to your care, and recognizing the differences between private practices and academic centers helps you decide what environment best fits your needs. Both offer advantages, and a second opinion can provide reassurance that your treatment plan is sound and aligned with the latest evidence.

Equally important is how you prepare for your consultations. Coming with a complete medical history, medication list, and organized records gives your oncologist a clear picture from the start. Asking thoughtful questions about diagnosis, treatment options, side effects, and long-term outlook not only helps you understand your care but also establishes you as an active partner in the process. Patients like Lydia show us that readiness empowers not only the medical team but also the patient, giving her a stronger voice in her care. The more prepared you are, the more confidence you will feel in both your treatment plan and your care team. By combining informed preparation with the right doctors in the right setting, you create the foundation for personalized, coordinated, and effective cancer care.

One final note before you move forward: The guidance in this chapter reflects what I have seen work well for many patients, and I offer it because I genuinely believe it will serve you well. **But** I also understand that a cancer diagnosis can be completely overwhelming, and not everyone is in the right frame of mind to tackle all of this immediately. If that is where you are right now, that is completely understandable. There is no perfect timeline, so give yourself the time that you need to be ready. Try to do what you can, when you can, and come back to the rest when you are ready.

Part II

Workup and Management

Chapter 4

From Scans to Staging: Understanding Your Workup

Navigating the initial phases of a cancer diagnosis can be overwhelming, but once you understand the process, it should appear more logical. In this chapter, I aim to demystify the process of diagnosis and staging, which can include a multitude of tests. Understanding the various diagnostic tools, the significance of biopsy and pathology reports, and the intricacies of cancer grading and staging will empower you to be an informed participant in your care.

Understanding Radiology in Cancer Diagnosis

Radiology plays a pivotal role in diagnosing, staging, and monitoring cancer. Each imaging test has its strengths, and often a combination is used to get a more comprehensive picture. Below is a summary of some of the most common types of radiology used.

Common Radiology Tests in Cancer Care

When cancer is suspected or already diagnosed, radiology becomes one of your most important allies. Think of these tests as creating a detailed map of your body, showing not just where things are, but how they're behaving. Each test has its own superpower, and often your doctor will need more than one to get the complete picture.

Let's pause here. I know the number of scans can feel overwhelming. But understanding what each one does will help you feel more confident when your doctor explains why they're recommending a particular test.

CT Scan (CAT Scan)

A CT scan takes hundreds of X-ray pictures from different angles and assembles them into detailed cross-sections of your body, like slices of bread in a loaf. What makes CT scans so valuable is their speed and availability. Most cancer centers can do one within hours, and they show organs, lymph nodes, and tumors with excellent detail.

The test itself takes only five to ten minutes, though you might wait longer for preparation. Most cancer CTs require a contrast dye to be administered into the bloodstream intravenously (IV), and often, there will be oral contrast given as a drink. The IV and oral contrast help distinguish between normal tissue and areas of concern. You'll lie on a table that slides through a large donut-shaped machine. The radiation exposure is minimal but measurable, roughly equivalent to what you'd get from natural background radiation over two to three years.

PET Scan (Usually Combined with CT)

A PET scan is like adding a heat sensor to your body map. After a small amount of radioactive sugar called fluorodeoxyglucose (FDG) is injected into your bloodstream, the scanner detects where your body is using the most energy. This is why standard PET scans are often called FDG PET scans. Cancer cells are typically sugar-hungry, so they often *light up* on the scan, appearing brighter than normal tissue.

What that really means is this: PET scans excel at showing whether cancer has spread and can guide treatment decisions with remarkable precision. They're expensive and usually require insurance approval, but the information they provide is often worth the extra step. The radioactive tracer is safe and leaves your body through your urine within twenty-four hours.

PRO TIP: PET scans can give false alarms. Healing tissue, infections, and even inflammation from a recent biopsy can also light up. Don't panic if something looks concerning; your doctor knows how to interpret these findings in context.

MRI (Magnetic Resonance Imaging)

MRI uses powerful magnets and radio waves instead of radiation to create incredibly detailed pictures of soft tissues. It's particularly useful for imaging the brain, spinal cord, liver, pancreas, and reproductive organs. Some examples include breast cancer staging, evaluation of the extent of cervical cancer or a pelvic mass, and brain metastases, where MRI often provides information that other scans simply can't match.

So, a logical question would be: Why don't we always do MRI scans if they are more sensitive and don't use radiation? Here's the honest answer: While MRI excels at showing details, it also comes with trade-offs that make it impractical for every situation.

The first reason is time. MRIs take much longer, usually thirty to sixty minutes, compared with five to ten minutes for CT. When you need to fit multiple appointments into your day or when your doctor needs information quickly to make treatment decisions, that extra time becomes a significant factor. The machine can also feel confining (imagine lying still in a narrow tube with loud banging sounds surrounding you). If you're claustrophobic, talk to your team about options like open MRI machines or mild sedation with anti-anxiety medications.

Second is logistics. MRI is significantly more expensive than CT, and most insurance companies require prior approval, so factor in extra time for scheduling. There are also far fewer MRI machines available than CT scanners. If you need imaging quickly, or on a weekend or holiday, CT is often your only option.

Third, clinical appropriateness. MRI's sensitivity can sometimes work against us. It can detect small abnormalities that aren't cancer but still need follow-up, leading to unnecessary anxiety and additional tests. For routine monitoring or when we need a quick assessment, CT often provides exactly the information we need without the extra complexity.

Ultrasound

Ultrasound uses sound waves to create real-time images, much like the technology used to see babies during pregnancy. It's completely safe, involves no radiation, and can guide biopsies with pinpoint accuracy. Ultrasound works especially well for examining organs in the abdomen, like the liver and gallbladder, the thyroid gland, the ovaries, and the uterus, as well as suspicious breast lumps.

One of the limitations of ultrasound is that sound waves can't penetrate bone or gas. Its accuracy also depends heavily on the technician's skill. But for what it does well, it does very well.

The bottom line: If you have dense breasts or are at higher risk, ask your doctor about these newer options. They're not available everywhere yet, but they're expanding rapidly.

Bone Imaging

Traditional **bone scans** use an intravenously administered tracer that accumulates in areas where bone is being rebuilt or repaired. If cancer has spread to the bones, these areas often light up. However, arthritis, old fractures, and infections can also cause bright spots, leading to false alarms.

Increasingly, PET scans are replacing bone scans because they can show both bone and organ involvement in a single test. For monitoring bone health during treatment, **DEXA scans** measure bone density and help prevent fractures, especially important for patients on hormone-blocking therapies.

Mammogram (Overview: More Detail Below)

A mammogram is a specialized X-ray designed specifically for breast tissue. It remains the gold standard for breast cancer screening and can often detect tumors before they can be felt during a physical exam. Having a routine screening mammogram annually can catch cancers early and save lives.

Mammograms use low-dose X-rays and require breast compression to spread the tissue for optimal imaging. Let's be honest about the downsides. The compression is uncomfortable, sometimes quite uncomfortable, but it only lasts a few seconds and is necessary for clear, accurate pictures. The radiation exposure is minimal and considered safe for routine screening.

One important limitation is that mammograms can be more challenging to interpret in women with dense breast tissue, where normal tissue and potential cancers can look similar on the images. If you have dense breasts, your radiologist may recommend additional imaging tests for a complete evaluation.

Most women should begin annual mammograms at age forty, though screening recommendations may vary based on your individual risk factors and family history.

Which Scan Is Best: CT or PET?

The answer is neither, or both! I like to try answering this question with some patient examples because I think it will make the most sense in the context of real medical cases.

Patient Spotlight: Emily

Emily had just undergone major surgery for ovarian cancer. She and her husband came to me for a second opinion and were frustrated that her doctor recommended a CT instead of a PET scan. Friends and family insisted PET was the better test, and Emily wondered if she was missing something important.

Patient Spotlight: Anna

Anna, a lawyer with newly diagnosed metastatic breast cancer, was reluctant to have a PET scan at all. She worried that the radioactive sugar used in the test might feed her cancer or even cause another one to grow.

Patient Spotlight: Lydia

Lydia was only forty-five when she was diagnosed with aggressive triple-negative breast cancer. Her tumor was large, her lymph nodes were involved, and before starting chemotherapy, her doctor needed to know if the cancer had spread further.

Most of the time in these scenarios, the real issue at hand isn't the doctor's decision to recommend a CT scan or a PET scan; it's about the doctor not effectively communicating the reasoning behind their choice and missing a valuable opportunity to educate the patient. The lack of understanding leads to anxiety and often mistrust.

My favorite analogy to explain the difference between a CT and a PET scan is with a weather map showing a heat wave moving across a region.

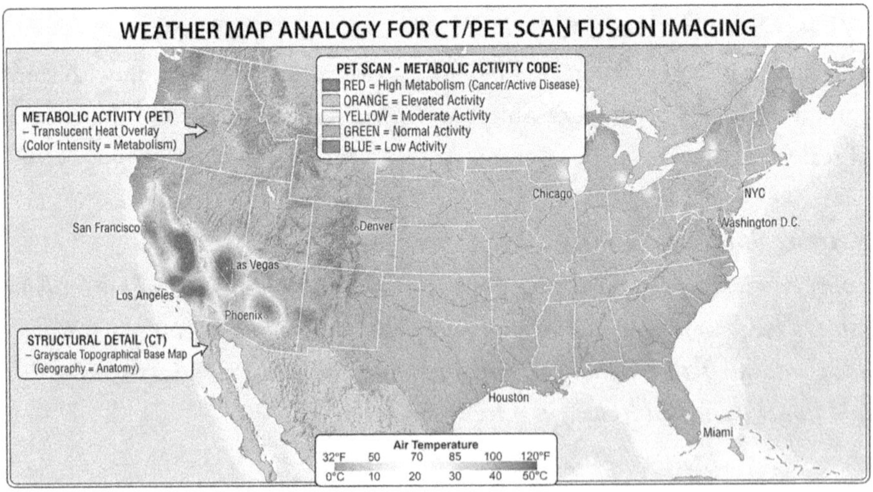

Imagine you're looking at a weather map that shows a heat wave moving across the country. The *geography* map gives you a clear picture of where the heat wave is, how extensive it is, and which areas are affected. This is similar to what we see with a CT scan. A CT scan provides us with a very detailed picture of the inside of the body. It shows us the structures of your organs and tissues in great detail, just like the weather map shows the geography, such as cities, states, mountains, and rivers. We can see the size, shape, and location of any abnormalities, such as tumors, just as you can see which areas are hardest hit by the heat wave.

Now, let's add another layer to our weather map. Instead of just showing where the heat wave is, it also shows us the temperature variations within the heat wave, highlighting areas where the temperatures are exceptionally high. This is like a PET scan, which doesn't really show us the physical structures, but instead shows activity levels in your tissues and organs. By using a special dye that contains radioactive glucose (sugar), a PET scan highlights areas where cells are more active. These areas *light up* on the scan, meaning they appear brighter because the cancer cells are using more sugar than normal cells—just as the hottest spots on the weather map glow with deeper color.

In real-time usage, a PET scan requires at least a basic CT scan as an underlayer so we can localize areas of activity (bright spots) to an exact place in the body, such as a lymph node, or to an organ like the liver or the bone. When we combine these two types of scans, it's like having a comprehensive weather report that not only tells you where the heat wave is but also shows you the intensity of the heat within it. In medical terms, combining a CT scan with a PET scan gives us a complete picture of the cancer's location and how actively it is growing. As you can see, CT scans and PET scans have a complementary nature in diagnosing and monitoring cancer. They offer different information, and at times, a CT scan can offer more important information if we are looking to see if a tumor has gotten physically larger or smaller in response to treatment.

Returning to Our Patients

Patient Spotlight: Emily

For Emily, who had surgery just three weeks earlier, a PET scan would have been misleading because all the healing tissue in her abdomen would have lit up. What she truly needed was a CT scan to show a clear, accurate baseline after surgery. Once she understood that, she felt more confident in moving forward.

Patient Spotlight: Anna

Anna's concern was very different. She was frightened by the idea of radioactive sugar feeding her cancer. Learning that the tracer leaves the body quickly, and that the PET scan was the best way to follow her bone disease, gave her the reassurance she needed. She agreed to the test, knowing it would help guide her care.

Patient Spotlight: Lydia

Lydia's situation carried its own kind of weight. At forty-five, facing aggressive triple-negative breast cancer, she needed to know whether her disease had already spread. Her PET scan gave her that answer—no distant spread—and cleared the way for chemotherapy.

Each of these women faced a moment of doubt about which scan was right. The real lesson isn't about choosing CT or PET; it's about the power of explanation. When patients understand the *why* behind a decision, tests stop feeling like arbitrary orders and start feeling like tools they can trust.

Making Imaging Work for You

The goal isn't to become an expert in radiology; it's to understand enough so that when your doctor explains their recommendations, you feel informed and confident in the plan ahead.

PRO TIP: If you do not understand why a particular scan was ordered over a different one, please ask your physician. Sometimes scans will be chosen in a particular order due to insurance restrictions. For example, some insurance companies will not approve a PET scan but will approve a CT scan plus a bone scan before they will approve a PET scan. Other times, a particular scan type may be ordered by your physician for a reason you do not understand, so make sure to ask.

To help you stay organized throughout all of your scans, the companion workbook includes two helpful tracking tools:

WORKBOOK CHECKPOINT: My Scan Timeline is a quick reference for logging all your imaging tests at a glance on page 4/1. Use **Individual Scan Results Pages** for recording detailed findings from each scan on page 4/2.

These tools ensure nothing gets lost in the shuffle and give you a clear picture of your progress over time.

A More Detailed Look at Breast Radiology

Mammography is a specialized type of X-ray designed for the breast. Its main purpose is early detection of breast cancer, often before a lump can be felt. There are several forms of mammography and related breast imaging tests, each with its own strengths and limitations. Which test is most appropriate depends on your age, breast density, medical history, and whether you are being screened routinely or evaluated for a specific problem.

Screening Mammogram

Screening mammograms are the routine breast X-rays performed in women who have no symptoms. The goal is to find cancers early, when treatment is most effective. Usually, two images of each breast are taken. If the tissue is dense, or if the images are unclear, the radiologist may recommend additional tests such as an ultrasound or MRI to provide more information.

Breast Ultrasound

Breast ultrasound, also called sonography, uses sound waves to create pictures of the inside of the breast. It does not involve radiation and is safe even during pregnancy. Ultrasound is often used to clarify mammogram findings, to evaluate women with dense breast tissue, or to guide biopsies. Its accuracy can vary depending on the skill of the technician, but it can be an important companion test to mammography.

Diagnostic Mammogram

A diagnostic mammogram is performed when there is a specific concern, such as a lump, nipple discharge, skin change, or when a screening mammogram shows something suspicious. The test takes more images from different angles and sometimes magnifies a particular spot so the radiologist can study it more closely. This helps determine whether further testing, such as a biopsy, is needed.

2D Mammogram (Digital)

Digital mammography has replaced older film technology in most centers. The images are stored electronically, which allows the radiologist to adjust and enhance them for better viewing. This has improved cancer detection, particularly in women under fifty and those with dense breast tissue.

3D Mammogram (Breast Tomosynthesis)

Breast tomosynthesis, often called 3D mammography, takes multiple images of the breast from different angles and reconstructs them into thin slices. This layered view helps the radiologist look through overlapping tissue, making it easier to spot small tumors. It is especially helpful for women with dense breasts and has meaningfully reduced unnecessary callbacks, with recall rates dropping from approximately 10.6 percent with standard mammography to 7.2 percent with tomosynthesis in a large ten-year study published in *Radiology* (ecancer 2024). That same study found a higher cancer detection rate with 3D mammography and a significantly lower rate of advanced cancers, suggesting tumors are being found earlier (ecancer 2024). Tomosynthesis is now widely accessible, with 90.5 percent of U.S. breast imaging centers offering it (Fornell 2024).

Contrast-Enhanced Mammogram

One of the most exciting advances in breast imaging is contrast-enhanced mammography. This test uses an injection of contrast dye to highlight areas on the mammogram of increased blood flow, which are often associated with tumors. Unlike standard mammography, it is not limited by breast density, with sensitivity improving from 71 percent to more than 92 percent in women with dense breasts (Lewin and Jochelson 2017). It is also an excellent option for women who cannot tolerate MRI, with roughly 70 percent of women who have had both exams preferring it for its ease and absence of claustrophobia (Klenske 2025).

Its diagnostic accuracy is comparable to breast MRI at a fraction of the cost and with greater accessibility. In a prospective study published in the *Journal of Clinical Oncology*, contrast-enhanced mammography identified an additional 23.9 cancers per 1,000 women screened among those with elevated risk whose standard mammograms were negative (Patel et al. 2024). For women who experience claustrophobia, have metallic implants, or live in areas where MRI is not readily available, it offers a meaningful and well-supported alternative.

Breast MRI (Magnetic Resonance Imaging)

Breast MRI uses magnets and radio waves to create very detailed pictures of the breast without radiation. It is the most sensitive imaging tool available for breast cancer detection, with studies showing that adding MRI to standard mammography and ultrasound improves detection sensitivity from 93 percent to over 98 percent (Chen et al. 2021). However, this high sensitivity comes with a trade-off: MRI has a higher rate of false positives than other imaging techniques, meaning something can look abnormal on the scan but turn out not to be cancer after further testing. These false alarms can lead to additional procedures, anxiety, and cost.

For this reason, current American College of Radiology guidelines recommend MRI primarily for women at high risk, defined as those with a greater than 20 percent estimated lifetime risk. This includes women with BRCA1 or BRCA2 mutations, untested first-degree relatives of known BRCA carriers, a history of chest or upper abdominal radiation before age thirty, a personal history of breast cancer or high-risk breast lesions, or a strong family history of breast cancer. Women with extremely dense breast tissue may also qualify, particularly when combined with other risk factors, as dense tissue significantly limits the ability of standard mammography to detect early cancers (Yeh et al. 2025). For women who meet these criteria, MRI screening is recommended to begin as early as age twenty-five to thirty, typically in addition to annual mammography rather than as a replacement for it. MRI is also used in surgical planning for women already diagnosed, helping to assess the full extent of any disease before an operation.

FES PET Scan (Estrogen Receptor PET)

If you have estrogen receptor-positive (ER+) breast cancer, you may hear about something called an FES PET scan. FES stands for fluoroestradiol, which is a radioactive form of estrogen. This scan works differently from the standard sugar-based PET scan. Instead of looking for cells that consume a lot of sugar, FES PET looks specifically for cells that have estrogen receptors. The radioactive estrogen attaches to these receptors, revealing areas where ER+ cancer cells are present. The FDA approved this test in 2020 as an adjunct to biopsy for use in recurrent or metastatic ER+ breast cancer, and the 2023 NCCN (National Comprehensive Cancer Network) Clinical Practice Guidelines further recognized that it may be considered for ER-positive disease more broadly (Covington et al. 2023).

Why would you need this instead of a regular PET scan? Sometimes ER+ breast cancers, especially slower-growing ones, do not show up well on standard PET scans because they do not consume as much sugar. FES PET can find these cancers more reliably, with studies showing it correctly identified active estrogen receptors 95 percent of the time while rarely flagging areas that turned out to be cancer-free (Covington et al. 2023). It is particularly valuable for identifying bone metastases, where it has outperformed standard FDG PET (Cuzzocrea et al. 2025). Unlike FDG, which tracks sugar uptake, FES uses fluoroestradiol, a labeled form of estrogen, to show exactly where active estrogen receptors are located in the body. Studies have shown that this scan has led doctors to change their treatment approach in nearly half of patients where other scans left questions unanswered, making it one of the more impactful newer imaging tools available for ER+ disease (Cuzzocrea et al. 2025).

A Note on Thermography

Some women ask about thermography, which uses an infrared camera to measure heat patterns on the skin of the breast. The idea is that cancer cells create extra blood flow and show up as hot spots that *light up*. While the concept sounds appealing, with no radiation and no compression, thermography has not been shown to be reliable as a standalone screening tool. A systematic review of twenty-two studies found a false positive rate of nearly 28 percent, meaning more than one in four women without cancer received a false alarm, while the test still missed a meaningful number of true cancers (Goñi-Arana, Pérez-Martín, and Díez 2024). The FDA has stated that it is not aware of any scientific evidence supporting thermography as an alternative to mammography, and thermography devices have only been cleared for use alongside proven screening methods, not as a replacement for them (US Food and Drug Administration 2021). For now, mammograms, especially digital 2D and 3D, remain the standard of care for screening and early detection.

Breast imaging has become more sophisticated over the years, offering women more accurate and personalized options than ever before. Screening mammograms remain the cornerstone of early detection, while diagnostic mammograms, ultrasound, and MRI provide additional tools when more detail is needed. For women with dense breasts, digital and 3D mammography often give clearer results. Newer methods, like contrast-enhanced mammography, have expanded the options for sensitive testing, and they rival breast MRI for accuracy. And while alternatives such as thermography may be marketed as appealing, they have not proven reliable.

What matters most is that you understand the purpose of each test, ask questions, and feel comfortable with the plan your doctor recommends. Knowing how these imaging tools work can help transform a confusing part of cancer care into a process that feels informed, intentional, and under your control.

Now, while radiological imaging gives us the map, the pictures are not enough to make a diagnosis (yet). To know for certain what we are dealing with, we need a biopsy. In this next section, we will review how we obtain a tiny sample of tissue from the suspected tumor to confirm a diagnosis.

A Closer Look at Biopsies and the Pathology Report

In the complex journey of cancer diagnosis and treatment, the biopsy is one of the most important steps. Often, an oncologist cannot even begin planning treatment until there is a biopsy showing cancer. A biopsy means removing a sample of the suspicious tissue so it can be studied under a microscope by a pathologist, a doctor who specializes in identifying disease.

The pathologist looks closely at the cells, including their shape, size, and arrangement. Additional special tests may also be performed on the tissue to learn more about the type of cancer, its growth rate, and even whether it carries specific genetic changes. This information is crucial because cancer is not one single disease. Cancer is many different diseases, each with its own characteristics and behavior. By understanding exactly what kind of cancer is present and how aggressive it appears to be, doctors can tailor the treatment plan to fit that individual situation.

Knowing how biopsies are performed and how pathology reports are written can help you better understand your diagnosis and participate actively in discussions with your care team.

Ways in Which a Biopsy Is Performed

Biopsies can be done in several ways, depending on where the suspected cancer is located, how accessible it is, and how much tissue is needed.

Fine Needle Aspiration (FNA)

An FNA uses a very thin needle, similar to the one used for a routine blood draw, to remove a small number of cells. It is quick and minimally invasive and can help answer the question of whether cancer is present. However, because the sample is small, it sometimes doesn't provide enough information for a full diagnosis.

Core Needle Biopsy

This type of biopsy uses a slightly larger needle to remove a tiny cylinder, or *core*, of tissue. Because it provides more tissue than an FNA, the pathologist can see not only the cells but also how they are arranged within the tissue. This makes it more informative than an aspiration in many situations.

Incisional Biopsy

With an incisional biopsy, a surgeon removes just a portion of the suspicious lump or tumor. This approach is used when the mass is too large to remove completely in one step. It provides enough tissue for the pathologist to study while leaving the rest of the tumor in place until a treatment plan is made.

Excisional Biopsy

An excisional biopsy removes the entire tumor or abnormal area, often along with a rim of normal tissue around it. This is more common when the lump is small and easily accessible, such as a breast lump just under the skin. It gives the pathologist the clearest picture because they can examine the entire area.

Endoscopic Biopsy

Some tumors are inside hollow organs like the lung, esophagus, stomach, or colon. In these cases, doctors use an endoscope—a thin, flexible tube with a light and camera—to look directly at the abnormal area and take tissue samples.

Image-Guided Biopsy

Sometimes the suspicious area cannot be felt or seen directly, such as a spot deep in the lung or liver. In those cases, imaging techniques like ultrasound, CT, or MRI are used to guide the needle precisely into the abnormal area. This allows doctors to obtain tissue safely from places that would otherwise be difficult to reach.

Liquid Biopsy

Liquid biopsy is a newer method that involves a simple blood draw. It looks for cancer cells or fragments of DNA that tumors release into the bloodstream. This approach is less invasive than traditional biopsies and can sometimes provide valuable information, especially for cancers that are hard to reach. However, because the amount of tumor material in the blood is often very small, liquid biopsies may not always give as much information as a sample taken directly from the tumor itself. I'll explain this topic in more depth in Chapter 5.

Pathology Basics

Once the tissue sample is taken, the real detective work begins. In this section, we will explore some of the basic components of a pathology report and what they mean. When a pathologist receives the tissue from the biopsy, they examine the cells under the microscope and produce a pathology report—a document packed with details that guide nearly every treatment decision.

The Grade and Stage of Cancer

When we talk about cancer, two important concepts help us understand and describe how serious it is and how best to treat it: grade and stage.

Grade

Think of the grade of a cancer as a way to describe what the cancer cells look like under a microscope compared to normal, healthy cells. It gives us clues about how quickly the cancer might grow and spread. Cancers are graded on a continuum from low to high. Sometimes a numerical system from one to three is used, with three being high grade.

Low Grade: These cancer cells look a lot like normal cells. They tend to grow slowly and are less likely to spread. This can also be referred to as *well-differentiated.*

High Grade: These cells look very different from normal cells. They usually grow more quickly and are more likely to spread. This can also be called *poorly differentiated.*

So, the grade helps us predict the cancer's behavior and aggressiveness based on how it appears under the microscope.

Stage

The stage of cancer describes both the amount of cancer in the body and how far it has spread. You can think of it as a map that shows how contained or widespread the disease is. Doctors often use a simple scale from zero to four to outline this. Staging systems are cancer-specific, so details can vary by cancer type, but the general outline below holds true:

Stage 0: This is very early-stage cancer, often called *in situ*, meaning the cancer cells are still in the place they started and have not invaded nearby tissues.

Stage I: The cancer is small and confined to the place where it began. There is no spread to distant parts of the body. Lymph node involvement depends on the cancer type and staging rules for that cancer.

Stage II: The cancer is larger than Stage I and/or has limited spread to nearby lymph nodes, depending on the cancer type. There is no spread to distant parts of the body. What counts as Stage II varies by cancer, which is why doctors rely on cancer-specific staging guidelines.

Stage III: This is considered a locally advanced cancer. It may have grown into nearby tissues or spread to regional lymph nodes, but not to distant organs.

Stage IV: The cancer has spread to distant parts of the body. This is also known as metastatic cancer.

Staging involves radiology scans, biopsies, and sometimes surgery to see how extensive the cancer is. By knowing the stage of cancer, we are able to create the most appropriate treatment plan for you. **It is also important to know that the stage of a cancer does not mean how sick you are.** Two patients can both have Stage IV cancer, one with a lot of disease involving several organs and another with a single cancerous lymph node far from the original tumor. Both are Stage IV, yet their medical situations are quite different.

Bringing Grade and Stage Together

In summary, while the grade gives us an idea about how cancer cells look and might behave, the stage tells us about the size of the cancer and how far it has spread. Both are key pieces of information that help your healthcare team decide the most effective way to treat your cancer.

PRO TIP for understanding cancer types: A cancer is named by where it originated and not by where it has spread. If a patient has breast cancer and a tumor in the lung, the tumor in the lung is breast cancer metastatic to the lung and not lung cancer. This is an important distinction because, in general, cancers are treated by type, which is defined by where they started.

Pathology tells us not only what type of cancer it is but also how the cancer behaves. One of the most important clues comes from receptors and proteins on the cancer cells, which act like signals or switches that can drive growth—or become targets for therapy. Next, we will explore the meaning of a receptor and some of the common ones seen in pathology reports.

What Is a Receptor?

Receptors are proteins in or on cells that can attach to certain substances in the blood. I often describe them as working like old-fashioned TV antennas, searching for signals in the air. When the antenna picks up the right signal, it sends it into the television and produces a picture. A receptor works the same way. It picks up a signal from outside the cell, such as a hormone, and then sends instructions into the cell. Those instructions can tell the cell to grow, divide, or even die.

Another way to think about a receptor is like a lock on a tiny door on the surface of a cell. To open the lock, you need the right key. In breast cancer, one of the most important keys is estrogen. Estrogen fits into the estrogen receptor and unlocks the door, sending a message to the cancer cell to grow.

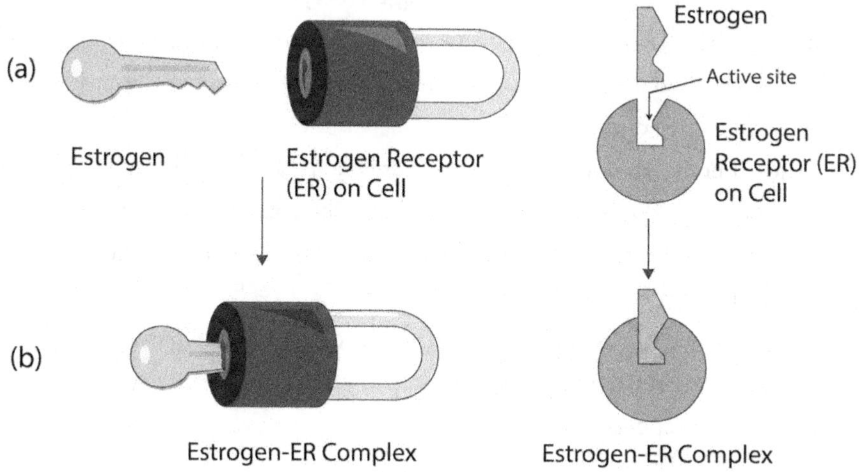

A mainstay in breast cancer treatment includes blocking the receptor. Treatments like tamoxifen are designed to mimic estrogen closely enough to fit into the lock but not open it. By blocking the receptor in this way, tamoxifen prevents estrogen from getting in and telling the cell to grow. For those of you with a science background, this is called a *competitive inhibitor*.

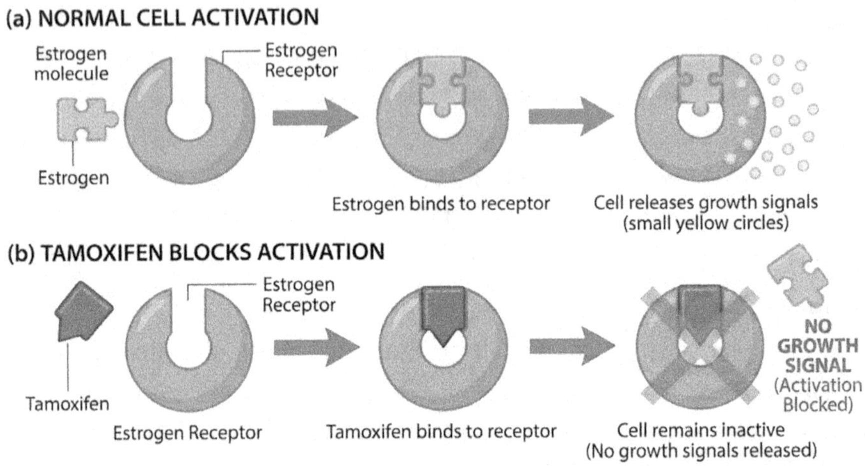

Breast cancers are often tested for **estrogen receptors (ER)** and **progesterone receptors (PR)**. Estrogen and progesterone can stimulate the growth of cancer cells that have these receptors. Different types of anti-estrogen therapy will be discussed in a later chapter.

The other key receptor in breast cancer is called **HER2**. HER2 is a protein that normally helps cells grow and repair themselves, but in some cancers, there are too many copies of it. When HER2 is overproduced, the cancer cells can grow and divide very quickly.

Unlike ER and PR, HER2 is usually reported in your pathology report with a score that reflects how many receptors are seen on the surface of the cancer cells after special staining:

- **0**: The cancer does not have extra HER2 receptors. This is considered *HER2-negative.*
- **1+**: The cancer shows a very low level of HER2. This is now recognized as *HER2-low* and may have implications for treatment.

- **2+**: This is a borderline or *equivocal* result. More testing is usually done to clarify whether HER2 is truly overproduced.
- **3+**: The cancer has a high level of HER2 receptors. This is considered *HER2-positive.*

HER2-positive cancers used to be some of the most aggressive breast cancers, but this changed dramatically once targeted therapies like trastuzumab (Herceptin) were developed. These medications specifically block HER2 receptors and have improved survival for many patients.

In summary, receptors are like antennas or locks on cancer cells. Whether your cancer has ER, PR, and/or HER2 receptors is one of the most important pieces of information in your pathology report because it helps guide treatment decisions.

Reviewing Your Pathology Report

A pathology report from a cancer biopsy is one of the most important documents in your medical chart. It contains the details that allow your doctors to confirm the diagnosis and guide treatment decisions. After a pathologist has studied your tissue under the microscope, they generate this report.

We reviewed the main sections above, but it may be helpful to see what a real pathology report looks like. Below are two examples of what a pathology report could have looked like for our patient, Jane. I've included annotations in plain language afterwards, so you can better understand what each part means.

Pathology Report—Example 1 (Core Needle Biopsy)

Patient Information:
Name: Jane E. Doe
Date of Birth: 05/08/1980
Medical Record Number: 987654321

Specimen Information:
Biopsy Date: 03/25/2024
Specimen Type: Core needle biopsy
Site of Biopsy: Left breast, upper outer quadrant

Clinical History:
The patient reported a palpable lump in the right breast during a routine self-exam. Mammography and subsequent ultrasound confirmed a 1.5 cm irregular mass. No previous history of breast disease.

Microscopic Description:
Microscopic examination reveals invasive ductal carcinoma characterized by nests and cords of malignant epithelial cells infiltrating the fibrous stroma. The cells exhibit high nuclear grade, moderate pleomorphism, and conspicuous nucleoli. Mitotic figures are readily identified.

Diagnosis:
Invasive ductal carcinoma of the right breast.

Tumor Grading:
Grade 3 (Poorly differentiated).

Tumor Staging:
Not applicable for the biopsy specimen.

Margins:
Not applicable for core biopsy.

Special Tests:
Estrogen Receptor (ER): Positive (90 percent)
Progesterone Receptor (PR): Positive (85 percent)
HER2: Negative (1+ by IHC)
Ki-67 Proliferation Index: 25 percent

Pathologist's Comments:
The biopsy is diagnostic of invasive ductal carcinoma, Grade 3, with positive hormone receptor status and negative HER2 overexpression. The findings suggest a hormone receptor-positive, HER2-negative breast cancer. Further staging is necessary to guide treatment planning.

Annotations and What This Means

- **Diagnosis:** Invasive ductal carcinoma is the most common type of breast cancer. It starts in the milk ducts and invades the surrounding breast tissue.
- **Grade 3:** These cells look very abnormal and are growing quickly. Grade helps predict aggressiveness.
- **Stage:** Stage cannot be determined from a biopsy alone. Imaging and surgery provide that information.
- **Margins:** Margins are often not reported on a biopsy. They are best assessed after surgical removal of a tumor.
- **Receptors (ER/PR positive):** The cancer depends on estrogen and progesterone for growth. This is important because it means anti-estrogen treatments can be effective.
- **HER2 (1+):** This cancer is HER2 negative, but the 1+ score is now sometimes referred to as *HER2-low*, which may influence treatment options.
- **Ki-67** (25 percent)**:** About one-quarter of the cancer cells are actively dividing. This suggests a moderate growth rate.

- **Pathologist's Comments:** The overall picture is a common breast cancer subtype: ER+/PR+, HER2-negative, high grade. This profile guides treatment decisions such as hormone therapy and possibly chemotherapy, but remember, we also need the stage of the cancer to make a complete treatment decision.

Pathology Report—Example 2 (Breast Lumpectomy and Sentinel Lymph Node Biopsy)

Specimen Received:
Left breast lumpectomy and sentinel lymph node biopsy.

Gross Description:

1. **Lumpectomy Specimen:**
   Received is an oriented lumpectomy specimen measuring 4.5 × 3.2 × 2.1 cm. The specimen is inked as follows: anterior (blue), posterior (black), superior (yellow), inferior (green), medial (red), lateral (orange). Serial sectioning reveals a firm, irregular mass measuring 1.8 cm in greatest dimension, located 0.5 cm from the nearest (anterior) margin. The remainder of the specimen consists of unremarkable adipose and fibroglandular tissue.

2. **Sentinel Lymph Nodes:**
   Three lymph nodes identified, measuring 0.9 cm, 0.6 cm, and 0.5 cm.

Microscopic Description:

- Tumor Type: Invasive ductal carcinoma, Nottingham Grade 2 (moderate differentiation).
- Histologic Features: Tumor cells exhibit pleomorphic nuclei, moderate mitotic activity (8 mitoses per 10 HPF), and tubular formation comprising 30 percent of the tumor.

Lymphovascular Invasion:
Identified.

Margins:

- Closest margin: Anterior, 0.2 cm.
- All other margins negative, >1.0 cm clearance.

DCIS (Ductal Carcinoma in Situ):
Present, solid and cribriform types, nuclear Grade 2 with focal comedo necrosis, spanning up to 1.5 cm.

Receptor Status (Immunohistochemistry):

- Estrogen Receptor (ER): Positive (90 percent, strong intensity)
- Progesterone Receptor (PR): Positive (70 percent, moderate intensity)
- HER2: Negative (1+ by IHC)
- Ki-67 Proliferation Index: 25 percent

Sentinel Lymph Node Biopsy:

- Total nodes examined: 3
- Positive for metastasis: 1/3
- Largest metastatic focus: 3 mm (micrometastasis)
- Extranodal extension: Not identified.

Final Pathologic Diagnosis:

- Invasive ductal carcinoma, Nottingham Grade 2, 1.8 cm, ER+/PR+/HER2-, Ki-67: 25 percent
- Associated DCIS, nuclear Grade 2 with focal comedo necrosis, spanning 1.5 cm
- Margins negative, closest margin 0.2 cm (anterior)
- Sentinel lymph node biopsy: 1/3 positive for micrometastatic disease (3 mm)

Pathologic Stage (AJCC 8th Edition):
pT1c N1mi M0

Comment:
The findings indicate a moderately differentiated, ER+/PR+/HER2- invasive ductal carcinoma with associated DCIS. Sentinel lymph node biopsy shows micrometastasis in one of three nodes, without extranodal extension. Tumor biology suggests sensitivity to endocrine therapy. Clinical correlation and multidisciplinary team discussion recommended.

Annotations and What This Means

- **Gross Description**: The tumor was 1.8 cm in size and close (0.2 cm) to the anterior surgical margin. All other margins were widely clear.
- **Grade 2**: Moderately differentiated; between low and high grade in terms of aggressiveness.
- **Margins**: Negative, meaning no cancer cells were found at the edges of the removed tissue. The closest margin was 0.2 cm, which is adequate.
- **DCIS**: Non-invasive cancer was also present, spanning 1.5 cm. This is common alongside invasive tumors.
- **Receptors**:
    - *ER positive (90 percent)* and *PR positive (70 percent)*. The cancer depends on hormones to grow. This makes anti-estrogen therapies very effective.
    - *HER2 negative (1+)*. This tumor is not HER2-driven. With 1+, it is technically *HER2-low*, which may open new treatment options in the future.
    - *Ki-67 (25 percent)*. About one-quarter of cells are actively dividing, suggesting moderate growth activity.

- **Lymph Nodes**: Out of three sentinel lymph nodes, one contained cancer. The metastasis was small (3 mm), called a *micrometastasis*, and had not broken out of the lymph node capsule.
- **Pathologic Stage** (pT1c N1mi M0):
  - T1c tumor is between 1–2 cm.
  - N1mi Micrometastasis in lymph node(s).
  - M0 No evidence of distant spread.
- **Overall Picture**: This is a *Stage IIA breast cancer* by AJCC (American Joint Committee on Cancer) staging rules. It is hormone receptor–positive, HER2-negative, with one micrometastatic node. Treatment typically includes surgery, consideration of radiation, endocrine therapy, and possibly chemotherapy, depending on genomic (tumor DNA) testing and patient risk factors.

Pathology reports are dense, technical documents filled with medical terminology that can feel overwhelming. That's why your companion workbook includes the Biopsy and Pathology Report Organizer, which is a structured form that helps you translate your pathology report into understandable terms. You'll record your tumor type, grade, stage, receptor status, and other key markers in one organized place, with space to write down what your doctor explained and questions you still have.

In summary, as you can see, the cancer workup is not one single test, but a carefully coordinated process. Imaging shows us where to look. A biopsy gives us tissue to study. Pathology reports tell us exactly what we are dealing with, while grade and stage help us understand how aggressive the cancer is and how far it has spread. Receptor testing adds another layer, showing us what signals the cancer is listening to and which treatments may silence those signals.

Taken together, these steps transform the workup from a blur of confusing tests into a clear story about your cancer. That story is what empowers you and your care team to plan treatment with purpose and precision. The details may seem overwhelming at first, but remember—each piece of information is there to give you clarity, control, and confidence for the journey ahead.

WORKBOOK CHECKPOINT: My Biopsy and Pathology Report Organizer can be found on page 4/3. Don't worry if you have not had your surgery yet; just leave that blank for now. We will revisit it in Chapter 6.

Chapter 5

Everything You Wanted to Know About Genetics

Introduction: Why DNA Testing Matters

If you have been diagnosed with cancer in the past decade, then you are in the era of personalized medicine. Gone are the days when many types of cancer were treated the same way with chemotherapy or possibly hormone therapy. Now, there are so many nuances to differentiating cancers, and what follows is a myriad of treatment options available. Today, we can look at the DNA inside the cancer cells and often inside your own cells to create a treatment plan that's specifically designed for you.

Every cancer has a story written in its DNA. Some cancers develop because of inherited gene changes passed down through families. Others acquire these changes during a person's lifetime due to environmental factors, aging, or simply random chance. These DNA changes can take different forms. Sometimes it's a mutation, where one letter in the genetic code is switched for another, like changing a T to a C. Other times, a whole section of DNA might be deleted or duplicated. Think of it as if you were editing a book or a term paper, where sometimes a single letter is misspelled, sometimes whole sentences are missing, and sometimes paragraphs are repeated. By reading this genetic story, we can often predict which treatments are most likely to work and even choose treatments that will target specific abnormalities. This is personalized medicine.

And no, this is not science fiction! It's happening right now in cancer centers across the country. A woman with breast cancer might avoid chemotherapy entirely because her tumor's DNA profile shows it is not necessary. Another patient might receive a targeted therapy that attacks a specific weakness in her cancer's DNA. Yet another might learn that her family members need screening because she carries an inherited genetic change.

The tests that make this possible are broadly called genetic testing and tumor profiling. They're becoming as routine as blood work in many cancer treatments. But there is a lot of information to digest and understand. The reports are complex, the terminology is unfamiliar, and the implications can be life-changing.

In this chapter, we'll break down what these tests actually measure, when they're recommended, and how to understand what the results mean for you and your family. By the end, my goal is that you will have the knowledge you need to have informed conversations with your oncologist about all types of DNA testing.

Let's start with the basics.

The Role of DNA in Cancer

At the most basic level, cancer begins when there are changes or mutations in the DNA that lead to uncontrolled cell growth. These mutations can be inherited (germline mutations) or acquired during a person's lifetime (somatic mutations). Understanding these mutations has become increasingly more important in the treatment of cancer. In this section, I will explain the different types of DNA and how they are commonly used in oncology.

Genetic Testing in Oncology

Genetic testing involves analyzing DNA to identify mutations that may increase the risk of a person developing cancer. Genetic testing most frequently refers to germline testing for an individual, which analyzes the DNA that is present in every cell of your body. Through germline *genetic* testing, we are able to determine if the cancer is hereditary and if other family members might be at risk, thus providing the family with information that they can use to decide whether they want to be tested. Genetic testing for both the patient and any direct family members of the patient is important because the results will help to make informed decisions about preventative measures. Prevention can range from higher-level screening to surgery to remove organs at high risk of developing cancer. I always tell my patients and family members that knowledge is power and that the days of just *watching and waiting* should be left behind.

For the medical oncologist who is treating a patient for cancer, the results of genetic germline testing can also guide treatment decisions, especially in patients with genetic mutations in BRCA1 or 2 and other known genetic syndromes such as Lynch syndrome. Genetic testing is performed by isolating and examining the DNA from your own cells, which is usually obtained from a blood sample or a swab of the cheek. Currently, several commercial companies offer this service, but many cancer centers have also developed their own in-house testing services. These genetic tests can be ordered as specific sets for specific cancers or as multi-gene panels that include screening for mutations in dozens or even hundreds of genes. Please be mindful that not all genetic tests are considered medical grade and that some of the commercially available tests sold direct to consumers may not be accurate and could have false positives or negatives. I have seen several patients who used a very popular genetic test which suggested they had a BRCA mutation but, when re-examined by a medical-grade laboratory, simply was not there—so buyer beware!

Who Should Consider Germline Genetic Testing?

The decision about genetic testing has become much clearer in recent years, thanks to updated guidelines from major medical organizations. In 2024, the American Society of Clinical Oncology (ASCO) and the Society of Surgical Oncology (SSO) made their recommendations much broader and simpler (Bedrosian et al. 2024).

If You Have Been Diagnosed with Cancer

The new guidelines are straightforward. Anyone aged sixty-five or younger diagnosed with breast cancer should be offered BRCA1 and BRCA2 testing as a minimum. This represents a major shift from older guidelines that focused mainly on family history and age at diagnosis (Bedrosian et al. 2024).

For people over sixty-five with breast cancer, testing is still recommended in certain situations. These include having triple-negative breast cancer, being male, having Ashkenazi Jewish ancestry or another personal or family history that suggests hereditary cancer runs in the family, or being a candidate for PARP inhibitor therapy (Bedrosian et al. 2024).

Other cancers also have clear testing recommendations. The National Comprehensive Cancer Network (NCCN) recommends genetic testing for anyone diagnosed with triple-negative breast cancer at any age, ovarian cancer at any age, male breast cancer, pancreatic cancer, or metastatic prostate cancer (National Comprehensive Cancer Network 2025). Colorectal cancer diagnosed before age fifty also carries a strong recommendation for genetic testing under separate NCCN hereditary colorectal cancer guidelines (National Comprehensive Cancer Network, n.d.). The reason is simple: knowing whether these cancers are related to inherited genetic changes can help guide the most effective treatment.

Based on Family History

Even if you have not had cancer yourself, genetic testing might be recommended based on your family's cancer history. The strongest indicators include having a family member with a known cancer-causing genetic mutation, cancers diagnosed at unusually young ages, such as breast or colon cancer before age fifty, or multiple family members with the same type of cancer. Sometimes, one person having several different cancers can be a red flag, as can rare cancers like male breast cancer or ovarian cancer. Certain cancer combinations in the same family, such as breast and ovarian cancer together, also suggest the possibility of an inherited genetic change.

Most importantly, these are guidelines, not absolute rules. Your doctor may recommend testing even if you do not fit these criteria perfectly, or may decide it is not necessary even if you do. The key is that genetic testing has become much more routine and accessible than it was even five years ago.

Practical Considerations for Genetic Testing

Before you decide on genetic testing, there are a few practical things worth knowing. Most health insurance plans cover genetic testing when it is medically recommended by your doctor, especially if you meet the criteria we just discussed. If you are concerned about coverage, your doctor's office can usually check with your insurance company beforehand.

You will typically meet with a genetic counselor to discuss the testing process and the results. Think of them as your guide through the process. They will review your family history, explain what the test can and cannot tell you, and help you understand what the results might mean for you and your family. This is not a lengthy process, but it is an important step to make sure you are making an informed decision and understand what the results mean.

Some people worry about genetic discrimination, but the Genetic Information Nondiscrimination Act (GINA), a federal law passed in 2008, prohibits health insurance companies and employers from using genetic information against you. While these protections do not extend to life, disability, or long-term care insurance, knowing your genetic status often helps more than it hurts by allowing for better prevention and treatment (National Comprehensive Cancer Network 2025). In my opinion, if your doctor recommends genetic testing, the benefits usually far outweigh any concerns. You will receive information that you need to make the best decisions about your treatments, your health, and often your family's health too. To make this easier, I created an organizational tool to help you track your consultations and results.

WORKBOOK CHECKPOINT: My Hereditary Genetic Testing Tracker can be found on page 5/1.

Tumor (Somatic) DNA Testing

Somatic DNA is also referred to as tumor DNA. The DNA is isolated from a sample of the tumor and undergoes analysis, looking for mutations or other changes in the DNA that are known to cause or contribute to the cancer's growth and survival. This process is often referred to as *DNA Molecular Profiling (DMP)* or *Next Generation Sequencing (NGS)*. I should offer a word of caution if trying to read these reports as a layperson. The reports generated from this powerful method of analysis can often be overwhelming to read for someone not educated in the myriad of oncogenes that are often revealed. So, although I am a passionate supporter of my patients understanding their cancer and treatments, the tumor DNA analysis is at a higher molecular level than most of the other topics we have discussed previously. Therefore, as a starter, I recommend that when you review the report with your oncologist, you ask them to highlight what the most important genes in your report are and why they are important.

When Tumor DNA Testing Is Ordered

Your oncologist will typically order tumor DNA testing in several situations, so understanding when and why can help you know what to expect.

- **At Initial Diagnosis:** For many cancer types, tumor profiling is now routine. If you have been diagnosed with lung cancer, colorectal cancer, ovarian cancer, endometrial cancer, or advanced breast cancer, your doctor will almost certainly order DNA testing of your tumor. The goal is to look for mutations that can be targeted with specific therapies. For example, if you have lung cancer and your tumor has an EGFR (epidermal growth factor receptor) mutation, you might be eligible for targeted pills instead of traditional chemotherapy. Another very common example is ovarian cancer, where testing for BRCA1/2 and HRD (Homologous Recombination Deficiency) in the tumor will help determine if a PARP (poly-ADP ribose polymerase enzyme) inhibitor will be recommended for maintenance therapy. We will discuss PARP inhibitors in further detail in Chapter 7.

- **When Standard Treatment Is Not Working:** If a cancer has progressed despite treatment, your oncologist might order repeat tumor testing. Cancers can acquire new mutations over time, and these changes might open the door to different treatment options. This is particularly common in advanced cancers, where multiple treatment lines may be needed.
- **For Treatment Selection:** Several specialized tests analyze a tumor's genetic signature and help guide treatment decisions across different cancer types. These tests are different from the mutation-hunting tests we discussed earlier. Instead, they look at specific characteristics or activity levels of genes in the tumor cells to predict how a cancer is likely to behave and respond to treatment. This is the topic of the next few sections.

DNA Repair Deficiency Testing: Finding Functional Vulnerabilities

Some specialized tests sit at the intersection between mutation hunting and prognostic testing. These tests identify defects in your tumor's ability to repair damaged DNA, and these defects create exploitable vulnerabilities that can be targeted with specific therapies. Understanding these tests requires a bit more biology, but it's worth it because they can open the door to highly effective treatments.

The BRCA Connection

BRCA1 and BRCA2 are genes that normally act as guardians of your DNA, producing proteins that detect and repair damage before it can lead to cancer. Their primary job is to fix the most dangerous type of DNA injury a cell can sustain: a double-strand break, meaning a place where both sides of the DNA ladder are completely severed, not just nicked or frayed on one side. Think of it as the difference between a frayed rope and a rope that has been cut clean through. A frayed rope can still hold; a cleanly severed one cannot. Your cells face these breaks constantly, from environmental exposures and the simple act of dividing, and BRCA1 and BRCA2 are the repair crew that splices them back together accurately. This repair process is called homologous recombination, and it is your body's most precise method for restoring damaged DNA.

When BRCA1 or BRCA2 are mutated and no longer work properly, this repair system fails. Your cells can still attempt to patch the breaks using a less precise backup system, but errors accumulate, and damaged cells are allowed to grow unchecked. This state, where the homologous recombination repair pathway is defective, is what doctors call homologous recombination deficiency, or HRD. It is most relevant in ovarian cancer and increasingly recognized in breast, prostate, and pancreatic cancers. Importantly, the same weakness that allows cancer to develop also creates a therapeutic opportunity: PARP inhibitors work by blocking the backup DNA repair pathway that these deficient tumor cells rely on. When both systems are disabled, cancer cells cannot repair their DNA at all and die, while normal cells, whose BRCA genes are intact, are largely unaffected.

BRCA1 and BRCA2 mutations can occur in two distinct ways—they are either inherited or they developed in the cancer itself.

- **Germline (inherited) mutations:** These gene mutations are inherited from your mother or father. You are born with the inherited mutation just like any other genetic trait. The mutation will be present in every cell of your body and is the reason BRCA mutations can raise your lifetime risk of developing breast and ovarian cancer, and why your blood relatives may be at risk as well.
- **Somatic (tumor-only) mutations:** These gene mutations developed only in your tumor cells, likely due to environmental exposures or random mistakes in the DNA during cell division. You did not inherit it, your children cannot inherit it from you, but your tumor carries it, and it can still qualify you for PARP inhibitor therapy.

As an illustration of these concepts, I would like to present you with two different patient scenarios:

Patient Spotlight: Sandra

Sandra was diagnosed with HER2-negative early-stage breast cancer, considered high risk for recurrence. Her oncologist ordered germline genetic testing as part of her workup, and the results revealed that Sandra carried an inherited BRCA1 mutation. She completed chemotherapy as planned and then was eligible for an additional year of targeted therapy with a PARP inhibitor, which has been shown in clinical trials to provide a significant decrease in the patient having a recurrence (Tutt et al. 2021). Without genetic testing, that treatment option would never have come up. Sandra's story illustrates why germline DNA testing is now recommended for all women with breast cancer aged sixty-five and younger, and why the results can matter well beyond the question of family risk.

Patient Spotlight: Maria

Maria was diagnosed with advanced ovarian cancer at age fifty-eight. Her gynecologic oncologist ordered germline genetic testing, which came back negative for BRCA1 and BRCA2 mutations. Maria assumed that meant BRCA was not relevant to her care. However, her oncologist also sent her tumor tissue for somatic testing, which revealed a BRCA2 mutation present only in the cancer cells themselves, not in her inherited DNA. This tumor-acquired mutation made her eligible for PARP inhibitor, which she went on to receive as maintenance therapy after chemotherapy, a treatment she would not have been offered had her doctor relied on inherited testing alone (National Comprehensive Cancer Network 2025).

Homologous Recombination Deficiency (HRD) Testing

What HRD Testing Measures

HRD testing specifically is primarily used in ovarian cancer, and increasingly in breast, prostate, and pancreatic cancers, to identify tumors with a broken DNA repair system called homologous recombination.

The HRD Gene Family

HRD does not describe a single gene mutation. Instead, it results from defects in any of several genes involved in the homologous recombination pathway. The most well-known members of this gene family are BRCA1 and BRCA2, as described above. But the HRD family includes many other players: RAD51, PALB2, RAD51C, RAD51D, BRIP1, and about a dozen others. When any of these genes malfunctions, the entire DNA repair pathway can break down.

Why HRD Testing Matters Beyond BRCA

It is important to understand that your tumor can test HRD-positive even if your BRCA genes are completely normal because the HRD test doesn't just look for BRCA mutations. It evaluates whether your tumor's homologous recombination repair system is working, regardless of which gene is causing the problem.

There are three primary ways that the tumor HRD DNA test evaluates for abnormalities:

1. BRCA1 or BRCA2 mutations (the most well-known cause)
2. Mutations in other HRD pathway genes like RAD51, PALB2, RAD51C, or RAD51D
3. Chromosomal scarring patterns that show the repair system has been broken for a long time, even if we can't identify which specific gene is defective

The test looks at all three. It generates a score based on the overall damage pattern in your tumor's DNA, which scientists call *genomic instability*. If your tumor shows extensive chromosomal chaos and rearrangements, that's evidence that the DNA repair crew hasn't been doing its job, whether or not we can pinpoint the exact broken gene.

In summary, HRD testing identifies tumors with dysfunctional DNA repair, not just tumors with BRCA mutations. This broader approach means more patients can benefit from PARP inhibitors.

Immunotherapy Prediction Tests

Mismatch Repair (MMR) Testing and Microsatellite Instability (MSI) Testing

These tests identify defects in a different DNA repair system—the mismatch repair pathway. This system fixes small errors that occur during normal DNA copying. These tests are routinely ordered for colorectal and endometrial cancers, and increasingly for other cancer types, including gastric and small bowel cancers. If your tumor shows MMR deficiency or MSI-high status, you are much more likely to respond to immunotherapy drugs like pembrolizumab. These tests have become so important that many cancer centers now test all colorectal and endometrial cancers automatically.

PD-L1 Testing is commonly ordered for lung cancers, cervical cancers, and some other cancer types to help predict response to immunotherapy. This test measures how much of a specific protein (PD-L1) is present on your tumor cells. Higher levels often correlate with better responses to immunotherapy drugs, though the relationship is not perfect. Your oncologist will use this information along with other factors to decide whether immunotherapy should be part of your initial treatment plan.

Tumor Mutational Burden (TMB) testing counts the total number of mutations in your tumor. Tumors with high TMB (usually greater than 10 mut/MB (mutations per megabase)) are more likely to respond to immunotherapy because they produce more abnormal proteins that the immune system can recognize. This test is used across many cancer types, particularly when standard biomarkers do not provide clear guidance about immunotherapy eligibility.

WORKBOOK CHECKPOINT: My Tumor DNA Testing Tracker can be found on page 5/2, to record mutations detected in your tumor, understand which ones can be acted upon or targeted, and track targeted therapies or clinical trials for which you might be eligible.

Specialized Prognostic Tests

While somatic (tumor) DNA testing hunts for specific actionable mutations, and DNA repair deficiency testing identifies functional vulnerabilities, there is another category of tumor testing that serves a different purpose. These specialized tests don't look for individual mutations to target with drugs or identify repair defects to exploit. Instead, they analyze patterns of gene activity to predict how your cancer is likely to behave and which broad treatment categories (chemotherapy, hormone therapy, immunotherapy) are most likely to benefit you.

Think of it this way—somatic mutation testing asks: What specific weakness in this tumor can I exploit with a targeted drug? DNA repair deficiency testing asks: Does this tumor have a broken repair system I can take advantage of? Specialized prognostic testing asks: How aggressive is this tumor, and will this type of treatment help?

Breast Cancer Prognostic Tests

Oncotype DX

Oncotype DX is one of the most commonly used genomic tests in the United States for early-stage breast cancer. It analyzes twenty-one genes in estrogen receptor-positive (ER-positive), HER2-negative breast cancer to generate a recurrence score between zero and one hundred. A low score suggests chemotherapy will not provide much additional benefit beyond hormonal therapy alone, while a higher score indicates chemotherapy is likely to help (André et al. 2022). The test is typically ordered for women with early-stage, ER-positive, HER2-negative breast cancer, where the decision about chemotherapy is not clear-cut.

It is important to know that the score cutoffs are not one-size-fits-all. For postmenopausal women, studies have consistently shown that a recurrence score of between zero and twenty-five means chemotherapy can safely be omitted, while a score of twenty-six or higher supports adding chemotherapy to hormonal therapy (Sparano et al. 2018), (André et al. 2022). For premenopausal women, the picture is more nuanced. Even with a recurrence score in the low-to-intermediate range, premenopausal women with node-positive disease showed a meaningful benefit from chemotherapy in a large clinical trial, suggesting that menopausal status must always be factored into the interpretation of results (Kalinsky et al. 2021). This is why your oncologist will consider your recurrence score alongside your age, menopausal status, and other tumor features rather than acting on the number alone (André et al. 2022).

MammaPrint

MammaPrint takes a different approach, analyzing seventy genes to classify tumors on a spectrum from *low risk* to *high risk* for distant recurrence. While MammaPrint is FDA-cleared for use in both ER-positive and ER-negative breast cancers, in clinical practice, it is primarily used for ER-positive, HER2-negative breast cancer with between zero and three positive lymph nodes. It is particularly useful for women with early-stage, ER-positive breast cancer where the traditional clinical factors send mixed messages about prognosis, helping determine whether chemotherapy can be safely avoided.

A low-risk result suggests the cancer is unlikely to spread to distant organs and that chemotherapy can generally be avoided without compromising outcomes (Cardoso et al. 2016). A high-risk result indicates a more aggressive pattern and typically leads to a discussion about adding chemotherapy to hormonal therapy. As with Oncotype DX, age matters here as well. In the large APHINITY trial, women over fifty with a low genomic risk result did not benefit from chemotherapy, while women fifty and younger with the same result showed a small but measurable benefit (Piccart et al. 2021). Your oncologist will always interpret this result in the context of your age and overall clinical picture.

Breast Cancer Index (BCI)

The Breast Cancer Index (BCI) focuses specifically on whether extended hormone therapy beyond the standard five years will be beneficial. It combines two different genetic signatures to predict both the risk of late recurrence (after five years) and how likely you are to benefit from continued hormone therapy (Noordhoek et al. 2021). Your oncologist might order this test around your fourth year on initial hormone therapy to assist in the decision whether to continue for five additional years.

WORKBOOK CHECKPOINT: Your companion workbook includes page 5/3, **My Breast Cancer Prognostic Test Results Tracker**, to record your scores, understand what they mean, and document the treatment decisions made based on these results.

Gynecologic Cancer Biomarkers

Cancer treatment has become increasingly personalized, and this is particularly true in gynecologic cancers, where specific biomarkers can unlock targeted therapies and guide treatment decisions. If you have ovarian or endometrial cancer, your oncologist will probably order several of these tests beyond the DNA repair deficiency testing we discussed earlier.

Ovarian Cancer Biomarkers

Beyond HRD testing for PARP inhibitor eligibility, several other biomarkers help guide treatment decisions in ovarian cancer. Folate receptor alpha (FR Alpha) testing determines eligibility for antibody-drug conjugate therapy, a newer class of targeted treatment that delivers chemotherapy directly to cancer cells expressing this receptor. HER2 status is increasingly being tested in ovarian cancer, particularly in certain subtypes where HER2-targeted therapies may be beneficial. For low-grade serous ovarian cancer (LGSOC), testing for mutations such as KRAS and BRAF helps guide treatment with targeted therapies that block these specific pathways. Adult granulosa cell tumors are tested for FOXL2 mutations, which are present in nearly all cases and help confirm the diagnosis. Mucinous ovarian cancers have their own distinct mutation patterns that may influence treatment decisions and help distinguish them from metastatic cancers that have spread to the ovary from other sites.

Endometrial Cancer Biomarkers

Endometrial cancer classification has evolved significantly with molecular testing. In addition to MMR/MSI status for immunotherapy eligibility, several other biomarkers provide crucial prognostic and treatment information:

- POLE mutations identify a subgroup of endometrial cancers with excellent prognosis, and patients with these mutations may be candidates for less aggressive treatment approaches
- p53 testing by immunohistochemistry identifies aggressive uterine serous carcinomas that require more intensive treatment strategies
- HER2 status is now routinely tested in uterine serous carcinoma, as HER2-positive tumors may benefit from targeted therapy
- Endometrioid endometrial cancers are often tested for mutations in KRAS, PIK3CA (a gene that controls cell growth and division), PTEN (a gene that controls the pace of cell division), and ARID1A (a natural tumor suppressor), which help refine prognosis and may identify candidates for targeted therapies in clinical trials.

WORKBOOK CHECKPOINT: For patients with gynecologic cancer, biomarker testing can get complicated quickly, especially when different results open different treatment doors. Your companion workbook includes page 5/4, **My Gynecologic Cancer Biomarker Testing**, to help you record which biomarkers were tested, what your results were, what they mean, and which treatments or clinical trials they may unlock.

Circulating Tumor DNA (ctDNA): The Promise and Reality of Liquid Biopsy

You have probably heard the term *liquid biopsy* mentioned by your oncologist or seen it in cancer news stories. The concept sounds almost magical: a simple blood test that can detect cancer, monitor treatment response, and catch recurrence early. This technology does represent a genuine breakthrough in cancer care, but the headlines often make it sound more ready for prime time than it actually is.

This section is meant to give you a solid, patient-friendly foundation so you can understand what ctDNA is, what it can realistically tell us today, and why your oncologist may or may not recommend it. We will go deeper into how ctDNA is used in monitoring and surveillance later in Chapter 14.

What Is ctDNA?

Circulating tumor DNA, or ctDNA, consists of tiny fragments of genetic material that tumors shed into your bloodstream. Think of it as molecular breadcrumbs that cancer cells leave behind as they grow, divide, and die. Unlike the larger chunks of tissue we examine in traditional biopsies, ctDNA represents microscopic pieces of the tumor's genetic blueprint floating in your blood.

When we draw blood for a liquid biopsy, we are essentially fishing for these genetic fragments among the much larger pool of normal DNA that healthy cells routinely release. The technical challenge is substantial. Imagine trying to find a few specific grains of sand on a beach, and you begin to understand why ctDNA testing requires such sophisticated laboratory techniques.

One important point that is easy to miss is that ctDNA testing is not just *one test*. Different companies and laboratories may use different platforms, different gene panels, and different ways of measuring and reporting results. That is part of the reason why results can sometimes feel confusing, even when everyone is acting in good faith.

What ctDNA Can Do Well Today

Circulating tumor DNA is most helpful when we already know someone has cancer and we are trying to learn more about what the cancer is doing over time. In those situations, ctDNA can sometimes provide information that would otherwise require an invasive biopsy, a long wait, or simply cannot be obtained safely.

One reason this topic gets confusing is that ctDNA testing can serve two different roles.

The first role is quantitative monitoring. In this approach, ctDNA functions like a trend marker. We follow the amount of tumor DNA detected in the blood over multiple tests and look for patterns. A rising trend can be a warning sign that the cancer is becoming more active. A falling trend can be reassuring that a treatment is working. A stable trend may suggest the disease is controlled. This kind of testing is most useful when we are looking at the direction of change over time, not just a single number.

The second role is qualitative mutation testing. In this approach, ctDNA testing is often called a liquid biopsy because we are using a blood draw to look for specific tumor mutations. Sometimes that mutation information can help an oncologist choose a targeted therapy. Sometimes it can show that the tumor has developed a new resistance mutation, which helps explain why a previously effective therapy stopped working and helps guide what to try next. This can be especially valuable when a repeat tissue biopsy would be difficult, risky, or slow.

Essentially, ctDNA can sometimes tell us how much tumor DNA is present, and in other applications, can tell us what mutations the tumor may be carrying. Both can be useful, but neither should be interpreted in isolation. The value depends on the cancer type, how much DNA the tumor sheds, the quality of the assay, and whether the result will change the plan.

The Limitations You Need to Understand

While ctDNA is exciting, it still has limitations. Understanding these limitations protects you from unnecessary anxiety, unnecessary testing, and false reassurance.

Limited Sensitivity for Early Detection

Despite exciting research headlines, ctDNA is not yet sensitive enough to detect early-stage cancers reliably. Small tumors often shed very little DNA into the bloodstream, making them difficult to detect even with advanced tests. This fundamental limitation is one of the reasons why ctDNA is not standardly recommended as a general cancer screening tool for healthy individuals and cannot replace an initial tissue diagnosis.

When doctors suspect you have cancer, a tissue biopsy remains the gold standard, and this is unlikely to change anytime soon. Currently, a liquid biopsy cannot fully replace a tissue biopsy for initial diagnosis because tissue samples provide crucial information about cancer type, grade, and cellular architecture that ctDNA testing cannot yet reliably determine. A pathologist examining actual tumor tissue under a microscope sees things that a genetic test simply cannot capture—at least not yet.

False results remain a persistent concern with ctDNA testing, just as they do with all medical tests. False negatives occur when cancer is present, but the test fails to detect it, particularly with tumors that do not release much DNA into circulation. A negative test can feel reassuring, but it does not always mean what people hope it means.

False positives present an equally troubling problem. The test can detect genetic changes from non-cancerous conditions, such as normal age-related changes in blood cells that can mimic cancer mutations.

This is one reason oncologists interpret ctDNA results in context. We consider your history, your exam, your imaging, your other labs, and the pattern over time. A single test result rarely tells the whole story.

Variable Performance by Cancer Type

The performance of ctDNA testing varies dramatically by cancer type, and this variability makes it difficult to apply the technology uniformly across all cancers.

Some tumors are *high shedders* that release easily detectable amounts of ctDNA into the bloodstream. Others are *low shedders* that may go undetected even when present and actively growing. Your specific cancer type, its stage, its location in the body, and your individual biology all influence how reliable ctDNA testing will be in your situation.

What works well for monitoring one type of cancer may not be helpful for another, and this reflects biology rather than any inconsistency in your care.

Lack of Standardized Thresholds

The lack of standardized thresholds remains one of the biggest current limitations. Unlike many established cancer tests, the medical community has not yet agreed on standard ctDNA levels that clearly indicate the presence of cancer or the need for treatment changes (Fusco et al. 2025). Different laboratories use different thresholds, platforms, and analysis methods, and no universal consensus exists on how to report results when a detected variant falls near the lower limits of detection (de Jager et al. 2025). Comparing values over time or between facilities can therefore be unreliable, especially when different assays are used.

Cost and Insurance Coverage

Finally, the practical matter of cost and insurance coverage cannot be ignored. Many insurance plans do not yet cover ctDNA testing for all applications, leaving patients to pay out-of-pocket costs that can range from hundreds to thousands of dollars per test.

When a test is ordered repeatedly, these costs multiply quickly. For many patients, the decision about ctDNA testing becomes not just a medical question but a financial one.

Why Many Oncologists Remain Cautious

You may notice that your oncologist approaches ctDNA testing more cautiously than some of the media coverage might lead you to expect. We are not resistant to innovation, but we are careful about the current state of the evidence.

Many studies are actively researching when and how ctDNA testing provides the most clinical benefit, but the current evidence does not yet support it as a replacement for established diagnostic methods in most situations. Our goal is to ensure that when we do order ctDNA testing, it will genuinely serve a purpose and guide your care.

The Future of Liquid Biopsy

Despite these current limitations, ctDNA technology continues to evolve rapidly. Researchers are investigating more sensitive tests, better testing methods, and improved ways to interpret results. The hope is not just *more testing*, but better testing that actually improves outcomes and avoids unnecessary harm.

I am optimistic, but I am also careful. In cancer care, excitement has to be matched with proof.

What This Means for Your Care

Understanding ctDNA's current capabilities and limitations helps you have informed discussions with your oncologist about whether liquid biopsy testing might benefit your specific situation. Currently, I feel that this technology works best as a complement to, rather than a replacement for, traditional cancer care tools.

Remember that the goal of any test is to improve your care and outcomes. As physicians, we are trained not to order tests unless the results will change what we are going to do. If you ever feel uncertain about why a ctDNA test is being ordered, it is fair to ask directly: Will this be covered, and how will this change my plan?

We will revisit ctDNA in Chapter 14, where I will walk you through how ctDNA is used alongside scans and tumor markers, how to interpret changes over time, and how ctDNA can sometimes help guide next treatment choices. Workbook page 14/3, **My ctDNA/Liquid Biopsy Tracking Log**, will also be introduced.

Chapter 6

What Surgery Choices Really Mean: A Clear Guide Without the Overwhelm

As you step into the treatment phase of your cancer journey, it is important to understand the landscape of possible treatments, how they relate to your cancer stage, and what each entails. As I have mentioned before, knowledge is power, and understanding this information can empower you and demystify the process ahead.

Understanding Cancer Stages, Timing of Surgery, and Treatment Implications

Cancer treatment plans are often determined by the type of cancer and the stage of your cancer, as discussed in Chapter 4. As a review, the stage is determined by the size of the tumor, its location, and whether it has spread outside of the original location and lymph nodes. Each cancer type and stage will be treated by specific pathways and options. The NCCN (National Comprehensive Cancer Network; NCCN.org) provides standardized guidelines for oncologists to follow for each type and stage of cancer. These standardized guidelines are updated at least annually. Sometimes it's worthwhile asking your oncologist to provide you with a diagram or drawing illustrating your cancer stage, because this may help you visualize how cancer progresses and why certain treatment approaches are preferred over others.

Surgery can be a primary treatment method for many cancers, aiming to remove the tumor and sometimes the surrounding tissue. The decision for surgery and its timing depends on the cancer type, stage, and location. In some cases, surgery is combined with other treatments, like chemotherapy or radiation, to ensure the most comprehensive approach. In other cases, surgery is not feasible or recommended because the cancer has already metastasized (spread), or if the patient is not healthy or medically fit enough to undergo a surgical procedure. It is not uncommon for surgery to be delayed when a complication arises, such as the development of a blood clot requiring the patient to take blood thinners or an infection that could prevent the patient from healing properly.

Surgical Treatment of Cancer

Surgery plays a crucial role in cancer treatment, often as the first line of defense for solid tumors. Depending on the cancer type and stage, surgery may be used to remove the tumor completely, reduce tumor burden before additional treatments, or assess the spread of disease. Below, we will review some anatomy of the organ and some of the most common types of oncologic surgeries categorized by cancer type.

Breast Cancer

Understanding Breast Anatomy

Before talking about surgery, it helps to understand the basics of breast anatomy. The breast is not just one uniform piece of tissue. It's made up of lobules (tiny glands that make milk), ducts (the small tubes that carry milk to the nipple), fat, and supportive connective tissue. Surrounding all of this is skin, including the nipple and areola.

The breast is also connected to a network of lymphatic vessels that drain into lymph nodes, especially the nodes under the arm (axillary lymph nodes). These nodes are important in breast cancer because they are often the first place cancer cells spread.

When we talk about breast surgery, whether it's a lumpectomy, mastectomy, or lymph node removal, it's these structures we are operating on. Having a mental picture of where they are and what role they play can make the surgical options easier to understand.

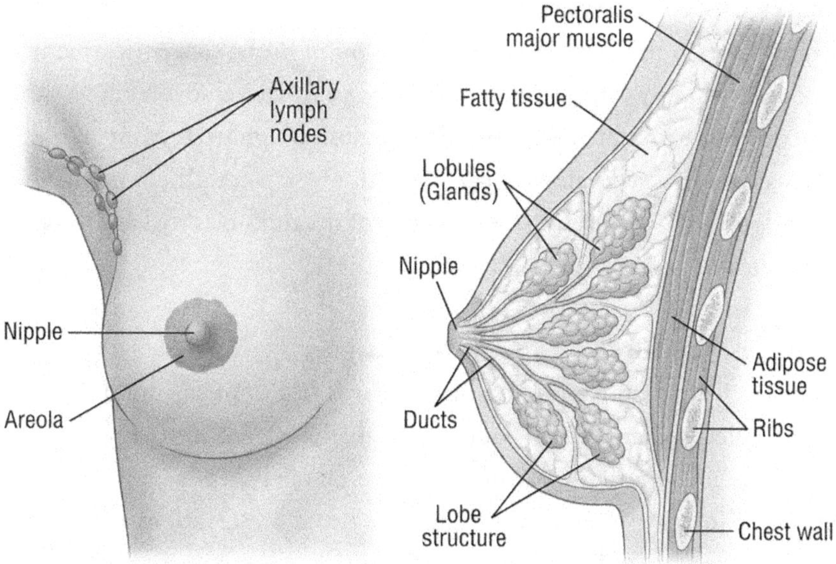

If possible, I think it is a good idea to do some preparation before you meet with your surgeon to discuss your surgical options, such as creating a list of important questions you want to ask.

WORKBOOK CHECKPOINT: The Pre-Surgery Preparation Checklist is on page 6/1 in Chapter 6 of your workbook. Please try to fill it out before your surgical consultation; it will be helpful. Once completed, you can file it in your binder under Surgery and bring the binder with you to the consultation.

Breast Cancer Surgeries

Surgery is often the first major decision point in breast cancer treatment. The reasons for surgery can vary. Sometimes the goal is to remove a known tumor, sometimes to avoid the need for radiation, and in high-risk women, to lower the chance of ever developing cancer in the first place. The type of surgery depends on the size, location, and biology of the tumor, as well as the patient's overall health and personal preferences.

Lumpectomy (Breast-Conserving Surgery)

A lumpectomy removes the tumor along with a rim of surrounding healthy tissue, called a margin. This option is usually offered in early-stage breast cancer when the tumor is small enough to be safely removed while keeping the breast intact. The major advantage is breast preservation, but it usually requires follow-up radiation to decrease the risk of the cancer returning in the breast. A lumpectomy plus radiation offers excellent long-term survival rates that are equivalent to mastectomy procedures in properly selected patients. The downside is that not all tumors are candidates, including some larger cancers, multifocal cancers, or when removing the whole tumor would leave a significant defect in the breast.

Modified Radical Mastectomy

A modified radical mastectomy removes the entire breast and the axillary lymph nodes, while leaving the chest wall muscles intact. Importantly, a sentinel lymph node biopsy is performed first; if those nodes are positive, additional nodes may be removed at the same time. This surgery may be recommended if breast conservation is not feasible, if the cancer is more advanced, or if a woman prefers to avoid radiation. It reduces the risk of recurrence in the breast, but it is a bigger operation with a longer recovery.

Skin-Sparing Mastectomy

In this procedure, the breast tissue is removed, but most of the breast skin is preserved, making reconstruction look and feel more natural. Studies show that it does not increase the risk of recurrence when used in carefully selected patients. The main drawback is that it is not safe if the tumor involves the skin or in inflammatory breast cancer. In addition, the preserved skin relies on a healthy blood supply, so smokers, diabetics, or women with prior radiation may face more healing complications.

Skin-sparing mastectomy is also most useful when reconstruction is performed immediately. For women not planning reconstruction, the benefit of preserving the skin is limited. Finally, while the skin is kept, the nipple and areola are usually removed unless a nipple-sparing mastectomy is specifically performed, which has its own criteria and limitations.

Sentinel Lymph Node Dissection (SLND)

Nearly all women with invasive breast cancer undergo a sentinel lymph node biopsy, whether they have a lumpectomy or a mastectomy. The sentinel nodes are the first to receive drainage from the tumor; if they are free of cancer, no further lymph node surgery is needed. The benefit is accurate staging with minimal surgery. The main risk is a small chance of lymphedema (chronic arm swelling caused by lymph fluid buildup), though the risk is much lower than with full node removal.

Axillary Lymph Node Dissection (ALND)

If cancer is found in the sentinel nodes, more lymph nodes may be removed in an axillary dissection. This provides important information and helps control regional disease, but carries a higher risk of complications, especially lymphedema. Because of this risk, ALND is reserved for cases where it clearly changes management.

Patient Spotlight: Jane's Story

Jane was in her fifties and post-menopausal when she was diagnosed with a 2.1 cm tumor in her right breast. Her cancer was estrogen receptor positive, progesterone receptor negative, and HER2 negative. Because the tumor was localized and operable, she underwent upfront surgery: a lumpectomy with sentinel lymph node biopsy. The good news was that the tumor was completely removed, although her sentinel node was positive. Still, surgery was only the first chapter. Jane went on to receive chemotherapy, radiation, and hormone-blocking medication. Her Oncotype test showed a higher risk of recurrence, so the additional treatments gave her the best chance of a long-term cure.

Jane's journey highlights how surgery often works in breast cancer: it can be the critical first step, but rarely stands alone. Each surgical option, including preserving the breast, removing it entirely, or sampling lymph nodes, is chosen carefully. Both the benefits and trade-offs must be considered as part of a larger plan designed to maximize survival and protect your quality of life.

Gynecologic Cancer

Understanding Female Reproductive Anatomy

The female reproductive system includes the uterus, cervix, ovaries, and fallopian tubes. The uterus is the hollow organ where a pregnancy develops and is also where most endometrial cancers begin. The cervix is the lower part of the uterus that connects to the vagina. The ovaries produce hormones and eggs, while the fallopian tubes carry eggs from the ovaries to the uterus.

In addition, the omentum, a fatty apron of tissue covering the abdominal organs, is often removed during cancer surgery because it is a common site where cancer cells spread. This is particularly important in the staging of ovarian cancers.

When surgery is performed, these organs may be removed in part or entirely, depending on the type and stage of the cancer. Knowing where they sit and how they are connected makes the surgical choices easier to follow.

ANATOMY OF THE FEMALE REPRODUCTIVE SYSTEM
(Cross-Sectional View)

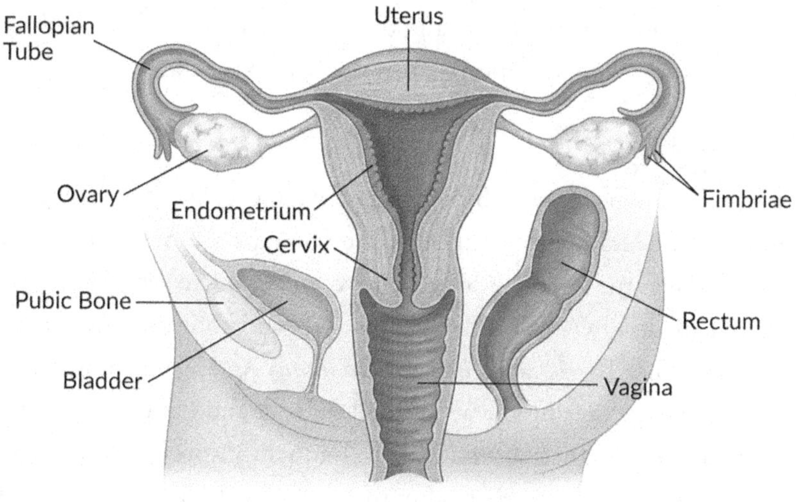

Gynecologic Cancer Surgeries

Surgery is central to the treatment of many gynecologic cancers, but the goals can differ. Sometimes the aim is to remove all visible disease, sometimes it is to stage the cancer accurately, and sometimes it is to reduce risk in women at high genetic risk. The type and extent of surgery depend on the cancer type, its stage, and whether fertility preservation is important to the patient.

Total Abdominal Hysterectomy with Bilateral Salpingo-Oophorectomy (TAHBSO)

This operation removes the uterus, cervix, both ovaries, and fallopian tubes. It is the standard surgery for many ovarian and endometrial cancers. By removing the primary site of disease, the surgery reduces the recurrence risk. For women with confirmed cancer, TAHBSO is often the foundation of treatment.

Robotic-Assisted Laparoscopic TAHBSO

This minimally invasive approach uses robotic instruments controlled by the surgeon. It requires only small incisions, often leading to less pain, shorter hospital stays, and faster recovery compared to open surgery. While outcomes are similar, not every patient is a candidate. For example, women with bulky tumors may still need a traditional open surgical approach.

Debulking Surgery

In advanced ovarian cancer, debulking surgery removes as much visible tumor as possible. The less cancer left behind, the better chemotherapy can work afterward. When the disease is too extensive for complete surgical removal at diagnosis, patients often start with chemotherapy and undergo surgery after the cancer has shrunk. This is called *interval debulking*. An omentectomy (removal of the fatty tissue covering the abdominal organs) and lymph node removal are also performed, since ovarian cancer frequently spreads there. Usually, additional chemotherapy is given after the interval debulking surgery as well.

Patient Spotlight: Emily's Story

Emily was diagnosed with Stage IIIC ovarian cancer. Stage IIIC is the most common stage at which ovarian cancer is diagnosed. The C is a subclassification of the stage. In ovarian cancer, this means that the cancer has spread outside of the pelvis to the abdomen (usually to the omentum), to lymph nodes, or to the surface of the liver or spleen. In Emily's case, her abdomen contained ascites (fluid in the abdomen that contains cancer cells) and multiple tumor nodules across the pelvis. Upfront surgery would have been unsafe and incomplete, so she first received three cycles of chemotherapy. Once her tumors had shrunk, her surgeon was able to remove all visible cancer at interval debulking surgery. Emily then returned to chemotherapy to complete her treatment. This sequence—chemo, surgery, chemo—is often described as a sandwiching of the surgery between the chemotherapy, and in Emily's case, allowed her to get the most benefit from both treatments.

Cytoreductive Surgery with HIPEC (Hyperthermic Intraperitoneal Chemotherapy)

In some centers, debulking surgery is combined with HIPEC. After tumor removal, the chemotherapy is warmed and then infused directly into the abdominal cavity. The heat improves drug penetration, and direct exposure bathes the surfaces where microscopic disease may remain. HIPEC is still not universally available, but in carefully selected ovarian cancer patients, it can improve outcomes.

Bilateral Salpingo-Oophorectomy (BSO) Without Hysterectomy

In some cases, the ovaries and fallopian tubes are removed while leaving the uterus and cervix in place. This may be done in premenopausal women with hormone-sensitive breast cancer, since removing the ovaries causes surgical menopause and eliminates estrogen production. Surgical menopause would be in lieu of the patient receiving monthly Lupron or Zoladex injections to suppress ovarian function. It is also used preventively in women with BRCA1 or BRCA2 mutations to reduce ovarian cancer risk. In some centers, patients at high risk of ovarian cancer may only have their fallopian tubes removed, since more recent research has shown that the most common site of origin of ovarian cancer may be the fallopian tubes (Kyo et al. 2020). The decision for this approach is made by carefully evaluating the risks and benefits of retaining the ovaries and preventing menopause in selected patients.

Cervical Cancer Surgeries

Surgery for cervical cancer depends on the stage, tumor size, lymph node involvement, and whether preserving fertility is important (fertility-sparing procedures). Each option has specific indications and trade-offs. A complete review of the staging for cervical cancer is outside the scope of this book as it is quite detailed, but an accurate description can be found at the Cancer.gov website (cancer.gov/types/cervical/stages).

Cone Biopsy

A cone biopsy removes a cone-shaped piece of tissue from the cervix. It is usually offered for early cervical cancer or when precancerous changes (often called CIN 2 or 3) raise concern for invasive disease. The benefit is that it can treat the problem while still preserving the uterus, which means future pregnancies may still be possible. The limitation is that if the cancer is larger than expected, additional treatment may still be needed. Because part of the cervix is removed, there can also be a slightly higher chance of pregnancy complications, like preterm birth, from the cervix being weakened.

Loop Electrosurgical Excision Procedure (LEEP)

LEEP is another fertility-sparing technique, most often used for high-grade precancerous lesions rather than invasive cancer. It is done in an outpatient setting with minimal recovery. The benefit is that it removes abnormal cells effectively while preserving fertility. Risks include incomplete excision (removal) if invasive cancer is present, and a slightly increased risk of preterm birth later in life if large portions of cervical tissue are removed.

Trachelectomy

A trachelectomy is offered to young women with small, early-stage invasive cancers who wish to preserve fertility. In this procedure, the cervix and surrounding tissue are removed, but the uterus remains. A cerclage stitch (a reinforcing stitch around the cervix) is placed to support future pregnancies. The benefit is that it allows a chance for childbearing after cancer treatment. The risks include higher rates of infertility, miscarriage, and preterm birth compared with women who have not had the procedure, as well as a small risk of local cancer recurrence.

Radical Hysterectomy

A radical hysterectomy is the standard for many women with Stage IB and select Stage II cervical cancers when fertility preservation is not a goal. It removes the uterus, cervix, surrounding tissues, and upper vagina, often with pelvic lymph node dissection. It offers excellent local control. The risks are loss of fertility, a longer recovery, and potential complications such as bladder or bowel dysfunction due to the removal of surrounding tissues.

Pelvic Exenteration

A pelvic exenteration is one of the most extensive operations in cancer care. It is considered only for women with recurrent or persistent disease when no other curative options remain. In this surgery, several pelvic organs may be removed, and new ways for the body to pass urine or stool are created, such as a urostomy (for urine) or a colostomy (to collect stool). It is a life-changing procedure with risks, but in select cases, it can still offer a chance for a cure when other treatments are no longer effective.

Patient Spotlight: Suzie's Story

Suzie is a vibrant thirty-two-year-old woman diagnosed with locally advanced cervical cancer after experiencing some pain and vaginal bleeding after intercourse. Her workup included a Pap smear, cone biopsy, pelvic MRI, and she was recommended to have chemoradiation. Since her disease was locally advanced and would be difficult to remove, surgery was not the first step in her treatment plan. Instead, she received weekly chemotherapy combined with daily radiation treatments. To help preserve her fertility potential, her ovaries were surgically moved higher in the pelvis, away from the radiation field, in a procedure called ovarian transposition. Surgery would only be considered later if her tumor did not fully respond. Fortunately, Suzie had a complete response to chemoradiation therapy and did not require surgery. She also retained her ovarian function and did not go into menopause. Suzie's case highlights an important principle in cervical cancer: the most effective treatment is not always surgery.

Final Thoughts on Surgery in Cancer Treatment

Surgery remains one of the most effective tools in cancer care. For some women, it is the first step toward a cure; for others, it comes later in the journey, after chemotherapy has reduced the cancer to a point where surgery is possible. And in some cases, surgery may not be the right choice at all. The decision depends on the cancer type and stage, overall health, and personal preferences.

What matters most is understanding *why* a particular surgical approach is recommended. Clarity on the goals, risks, and benefits allows you to move forward with confidence and a sense of control.

Consider these examples from my practice:

Patient Spotlight: Lydia's Story (Triple-Negative Breast Cancer)

Lydia, forty-five, had a fast-growing triple-negative breast cancer that was too large for immediate surgery. She started with chemotherapy and immunotherapy to shrink the tumor, then chose a bilateral mastectomy because genetic testing revealed a PALB2 mutation that increased her risk for future cancers. For Lydia, surgery was part of a larger, carefully staged plan, not a first step, but a pivotal one.

Patient Spotlight: Laura's Story (Endometrial Cancer)

Laura, a sixty-two-year-old teacher, was diagnosed with Stage III serous endometrial cancer. Her doctors recommended a total hysterectomy with surgical staging, followed by chemotherapy and immunotherapy. In her case, surgery was an important part of treatment because it removed the uterus, cervix, and nearby tissues where the cancer had spread. Even so, Laura hesitated. She worried about how she would recover, how the surgery might affect her daily life, and how she would face the treatment still ahead. Her story is a reminder that even when the medical plan is clear, the decision can still feel emotionally hard.

Together, these women show that surgery is not a one-size-fits-all solution. It may come at the beginning of treatment, later in the course, or not be part of the plan at all. The key is to see surgery as one tool within a larger strategy.

When you understand its role in your treatment plan, you can move forward with greater clarity, confidence, and calm.

WORKBOOK CHECKPOINT: Understanding surgical options is important, but putting that knowledge into practice requires concrete tools. Your companion workbook contains three helpful resources:

- Page 6/1, **Pre-Surgery Preparation Checklist**: Complete this before your surgical consultation to ensure you ask every important question, organize your support team with contact information, and prepare your home for recovery.
- Page 6/2, **Post-Surgical Recovery Planner Guide**: Use this daily tracking system in your Cancer Journey Planner to monitor healing, document symptoms, and catch potential complications early. Your surgeon will be impressed by your organized records. Set up your tracking system before your surgery date so you are ready to start documenting from Post-Op Day 1.
- Page 4/3, **My Biopsy and Pathology Report Organizer**: You should return to this workbook page to update any additional pathology you have obtained.

These three tools transform the concepts in this chapter into actionable steps. In the next chapter, we will explore the medical oncology side of the equation.

Chapter 7

The Medical Oncologist's Toolbox: Chemo, Hormones, and Targeted Therapies

As a medical oncologist, my main focus is on *systemic therapies*, which are treatments that travel throughout the entire body to find and destroy cancer cells wherever they may be. Unlike surgery or traditional radiation therapy, which target one specific area, systemic therapy works like a citywide transit system or the roots of a tree. Once the treatment enters the bloodstream, it can reach both the original tumor and any cancer cells that have spread elsewhere.

Systemic therapies come in different forms. Chemotherapy uses cancer-killing drugs that affect rapidly dividing cells. Immunotherapy helps your immune system recognize and attack cancer more effectively. Targeted therapies are designed to block specific weaknesses in cancer cells, such as a gene mutation or a protein they rely on to grow.

The goal of systemic therapy is comprehensive: to reduce the risk of cancer spreading, to treat cancer that has already traveled beyond its starting point, or to decrease the chance of it coming back. In many cases, systemic treatment works hand in hand with surgery and radiation as part of a coordinated plan.

WORKBOOK CHECKPOINT: Before we dive deeper, take a moment to fill out page 7/1, **My Systemic Therapy Overview**, in your Chapter 7 Workbook. This will help you organize the key details about your specific treatment plan as you continue reading.

Adjuvant Versus Neoadjuvant Therapy

Systemic therapy, meaning treatment that works throughout the whole body, can be given either before surgery, after surgery, or both. Which approach best depends on the type of cancer, the stage, and the unique details of the tumor itself. These systemic therapies may include chemotherapy, hormone therapy, targeted therapy, or immunotherapy, sometimes given in combination.

Adjuvant therapy is given *after* surgery. The goal is to wipe out any microscopic cancer cells that might still be hiding after the main tumor has been removed. Even if your scans look clear and the surgeon feels confident, the truth is we cannot see every single cell. Some of those invisible stragglers may remain in the surgical area, while others may already have slipped into the bloodstream or lymphatic system before the tumor was removed. Those are the cells that can later cause the cancer to return. Adjuvant therapy lowers that risk.

In breast cancer, for example, a woman might have a lumpectomy or mastectomy followed by chemotherapy, hormone therapy, or a targeted drug, such as a PARP inhibitor. These treatments are not chosen at random. The number of cycles and the drugs used have been carefully worked out through clinical trials, so there is usually a defined course to follow. Adjuvant therapy can also be **tailored, based on response**. For instance, if a patient has chemotherapy before surgery (neoadjuvant) and there is still cancer left in the breast or lymph nodes afterward, additional adjuvant therapy may be added to improve the chance of cure. In triple-negative breast cancer, this could mean a course of capecitabine (oral chemotherapy) or immunotherapy, depending on what was already given before surgery. In HER2-positive breast cancer, it could mean switching from trastuzumab to T-DM1 (Kadcyla). These are examples of how we, as medical oncologists, adapt the plan depending on how the tumor behaves.

Neoadjuvant therapy is given *before* surgery. The main aim is to shrink the tumor, making surgery easier and often less invasive. In breast cancer, this can mean the difference between needing a mastectomy versus being able to keep the breast with a lumpectomy. In ovarian cancer, we may use neoadjuvant chemotherapy when the disease is too extensive to be removed safely at the start. Another advantage of this approach is that it gives us real-time feedback. By watching how the tumor responds, we learn whether the drugs are working. If the cancer does not shrink as much as hoped, we can adjust the plan before surgery. Typically, patients receive a set number of treatments up front, but flexibility is built in.

Sometimes both approaches are used in sequence. A woman with breast, ovarian, or endometrial cancer, for example, might start with neoadjuvant therapy, then have surgery, and later receive additional adjuvant therapy. The choice of drugs depends on the type of cancer, the biology of the tumor, the overall health of the patient, as well as results from tumor-specific tests such as BRCA status or HER2 expression.

In Summary

Adjuvant therapy is about eliminating any cancer cells that may have been left behind after surgery. Neoadjuvant therapy is about downsizing the cancer (decreasing its size and extent) and, as an added bonus, showing us more about the tumor's biology and how it responds (shrinks or grows) to different treatments. Both strategies are powerful, and choosing between them is always individualized. It comes down to the cancer's biology, the evidence from clinical trials, and the goals for each patient.

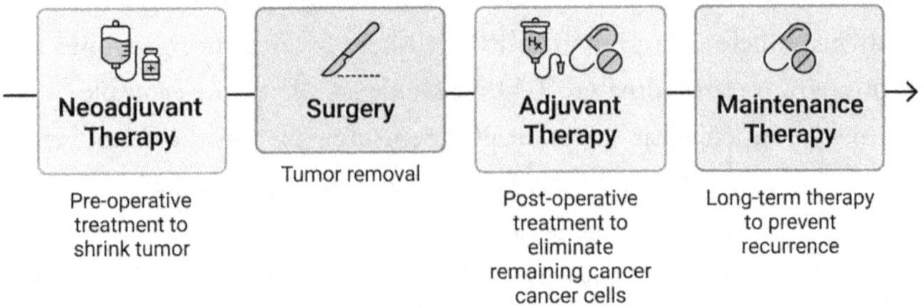

Patient Spotlight: Emily

Emily was sixty-two when months of bloating, getting full after a few bites, and pelvic discomfort led to testing that showed advanced ovarian cancer. A gynecologic oncologist reviewed her scans and examined her. The team obtained a biopsy to confirm the diagnosis.

Because complete removal of all visible cancer was unlikely at the start, Emily began neoadjuvant chemotherapy with carboplatin and paclitaxel. After three cycles, her symptoms improved, and her scans showed significantly less disease.

She then had interval debulking surgery where the surgeon removed her uterus, ovaries, and fallopian tubes, the omentum, some lymph nodes, and other visible tumor deposits. The operation was shorter and safer than it would have been without chemo first, and she did not need a bowel resection.

After she recovered, Emily finished the remaining chemotherapy cycles to complete her plan. Her follow-up included regular visits and attention to any new symptoms.

As you can see from this example, giving chemotherapy first can make a major operation more feasible and less risky, with better results.

Chemotherapy, Immunotherapy, Hormone Therapy, and Targeted Treatments

In recent years, the landscape of systemic cancer treatment has undergone a significant transformation. Beyond traditional chemotherapy, innovative options like immunotherapy and targeted therapies have emerged, offering new hope and tailored approaches to battling cancer.

Understanding Chemotherapy

Chemotherapy has been one of the cornerstones of cancer treatment for decades. These medicines work by interfering with cell division, making them especially effective against cancer cells, which divide and grow uncontrollably. Because chemotherapy drugs travel through the bloodstream, they can reach cancer cells throughout the body, not just at the original tumor site.

The challenge is that chemotherapy does not distinguish perfectly between cancer cells and normal cells that also divide quickly. This is why tissues like hair follicles, the lining of the mouth and digestive tract, and bone marrow (where blood cells are made) are often affected. Side effects such as hair loss, nausea, mouth sores, and lowered blood counts result from this impact on healthy, fast-growing cells.

Even with these challenges, chemotherapy remains one of the most powerful tools in oncology. For many cancers, it improves survival, reduces recurrence risk, and sometimes cures the disease altogether. It is also often combined with newer treatments, such as targeted therapies and immunotherapies, to improve results while personalizing care.

Understanding Hormone (Endocrine) Therapy

Hormone therapy, also called endocrine therapy, plays a central role in the treatment of breast and some gynecologic cancers. These cancers may depend on hormones such as estrogen or progesterone to grow and spread. By reducing hormone levels in the body or blocking their action, hormone therapy cuts off the *fuel supply* that drives cancer growth. You may recall that in Chapter 4, we discussed one way in which receptors may function like tiny antennas or locks on the surface of cancer cells that pick up signals in the blood from the body. When estrogen binds to the estrogen receptor (ER) on a cancer cell, it sends a message for the cell to grow and divide. In breast cancer, this receptor signaling can be a powerful driver of tumor growth.

Hormone therapy is designed to block this pathway. In other words, if estrogen is the *key* that fits into the receptor *lock*, hormone therapy either blocks the lock (tamoxifen), takes away the key (aromatase inhibitor), or destroys the lock/receptor altogether (SERDs, Selective Estrogen Receptor Degraders). This approach has been one of the most successful ways to treat hormone-sensitive cancers, especially breast cancer and certain gynecologic cancers.

Hormone therapy is generally less toxic than chemotherapy, but it often comes with side effects that can be difficult to live with day-to-day, such as hot flashes, joint aches, vaginal dryness, and brain fog. Despite these challenges, which can be significant and life-altering, anti-estrogen therapy remains one of the most effective ways we have to lower the risk of recurrence and improve survival in hormone-positive tumors.

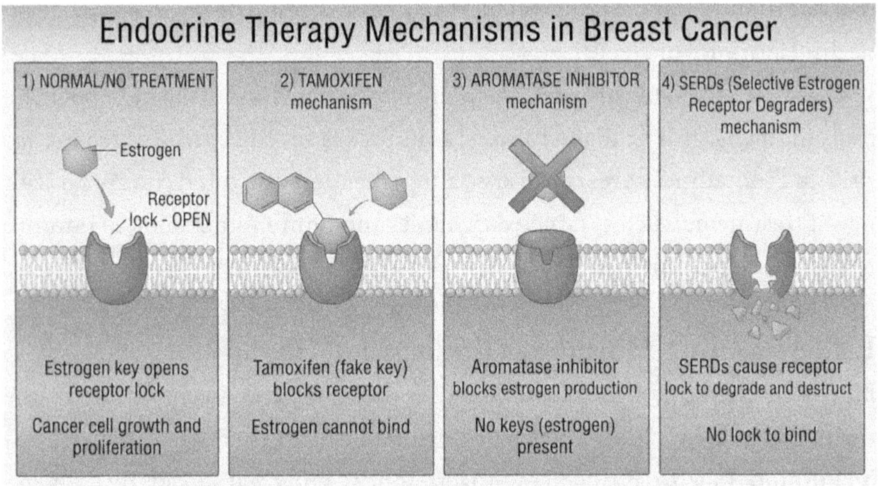

Selective Estrogen Receptor Modulators (SERMs)

Drugs like **tamoxifen** and **raloxifene** bind to estrogen receptors on cancer cells. They mimic estrogen closely enough to fit into the receptor, but without sending the *grow* signal. This blocks estrogen from activating the receptor and slows cancer growth in a process known as competitive inhibition.

Aromatase Inhibitors (AIs)

In postmenopausal women, most estrogen is made outside of the ovaries in other tissues, such as fat cells, breast tissue, and adrenal glands, by an enzyme called aromatase. Drugs such as **letrozole**, **anastrozole**, and **exemestane** block this enzyme, cutting off estrogen production almost completely. Without estrogen, the receptor has no key to turn on growth signals.

Selective Estrogen Receptor Degraders (SERDs)

SERDs not only block the receptor but also destroy it. The most established example is **fulvestrant (Faslodex)**, given as a monthly injection. New oral SERDs, such as **elacestrant**, have recently been developed, offering more convenience and better options for patients whose cancers stop responding to other hormone therapies when they develop a DNA mutation called ESR-1.

Ovarian Suppression

For premenopausal women, shutting down the ovaries removes the main source of estrogen, thus putting the patient into menopause. This can be done temporarily with injections (goserelin, leuprolide) or permanently with surgery (oophorectomy). Ovarian suppression is often used in combination with tamoxifen or an aromatase inhibitor to maximize effectiveness.

Progesterone Therapy

In certain **endometrial cancers**, progesterone therapy, such as megestrol acetate, can counteract the effects of estrogen and slow cancer growth. In younger women, this can sometimes be used as a fertility-sparing treatment instead of immediate surgery in lower-grade tumors. Currently, progesterone therapy is not frequently used in the treatment of breast cancer.

Impact on Fertility

Chemotherapy and hormone therapy can significantly affect fertility in younger women. Chemotherapy damages the eggs in the ovaries, and treatments like ovarian suppression or aromatase inhibitors induce menopause or severely reduce ovarian function. If you are of childbearing age and have not yet discussed fertility preservation with your oncologist, now is the time. Even if you've already started hormone therapy, options may still be available depending on your situation. Refer to Chapter 3 for a comprehensive discussion of fertility preservation, or speak with your oncologist about a referral to a reproductive endocrinologist.

> **WORKBOOK CHECKPOINT:** If your cancer is hormone-driven (ER+ or PR+), pause here and complete page 7/2, **Understanding My Hormone Therapy**. Use the decoder key to identify which type you're taking and note any side effects your doctor mentioned.

The Rise of Immunotherapy

Immunotherapy represents a true shift in how we think about cancer treatment. Instead of directly attacking cancer cells with drugs, immunotherapy works by helping your body's own immune system recognize and fight the disease.

Cancer cells are clever. They often disguise themselves so that immune cells pass them by, almost like a thief hiding in plain sight. Immunotherapy lifts that disguise. It *unmasks* the cancer so your immune system can see it as dangerous and attack it with precision.

How Immunotherapy Works

The most common immunotherapy used in breast and gynecologic cancers is called a **checkpoint inhibitor**. You can think of checkpoints as brakes on the immune system. Cancer cells sometimes take advantage of these brakes to hide from attack. Drugs such as pembrolizumab (Keytruda), nivolumab (Opdivo), and dostarlimab (Jemperli) work by releasing those brakes, most often by blocking the PD-1 or PD-L1 pathway.

Once those brakes are lifted, your T cells, which are the immune system's soldiers, are better able to recognize and attack cancer. This is why we often test tumors for markers such as **PD-L1** or **mismatch repair deficiency/ microsatellite instability**. In some cancers, these markers help identify the patients most likely to benefit.

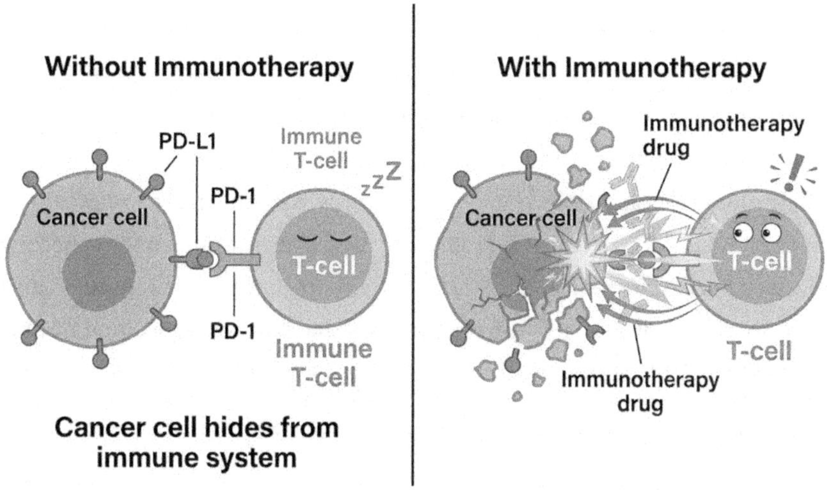

Unlike chemotherapy, which directly attacks rapidly dividing cells, immunotherapy works by helping your own immune system do its job more effectively. It does not work for everyone, but for some patients it can produce deep and long-lasting responses, even in advanced cancer.

Checkpoint inhibitors are now used in several cancers, including triple-negative breast cancer, endometrial cancer, cervical cancer, lung cancer, melanoma, and others. Depending on the type of cancer and its tumor markers, they may be used by themselves or paired with chemotherapy or other medicines to improve results. That is now starting to happen in some ovarian cancers too. For example, some women with platinum-resistant ovarian cancer may now receive pembrolizumab along with chemotherapy, which is an important reminder that cancer treatment keeps evolving, even in cancers that once seemed less likely to respond to immunotherapy.

Patient Spotlight: Maria

Maria was in her late sixties when she was diagnosed with advanced endometrial cancer. Despite surgery and chemotherapy, her cancer quickly returned and spread to her lungs. She and her family were devastated, as this usually meant that time was short. Genetic testing of her tumor revealed a feature called mismatch repair deficiency, which made her eligible for immunotherapy. Maria began treatment with pembrolizumab, and within months, her scans showed her tumors shrinking. Today, years later, Maria is still in remission. For her, immunotherapy transformed what seemed like a hopeless situation into a new lease on life.

Immunotherapy does not work for every patient or every cancer type, and it can sometimes cause side effects when the immune system becomes *too active* and attacks healthy tissues. But when it works, the results can be impressive and can change the outlook for patients in ways we could not have imagined a decade ago.

WORKBOOK CHECKPOINT: If you're receiving immunotherapy, turn to page 7/3, **Section B: If I'm On Immunotherapy**, to track your medication and understand which side effects require immediate attention. Immunotherapy side effects can affect any organ, so knowing what to watch for is critical.

The Precision of Targeted Therapies

Targeted therapy is one of the most interesting and exciting parts of modern oncology. It focuses on specific genes, proteins, or cellular pathways that drive cancer growth and survival. Unlike chemotherapy, which affects all rapidly dividing cells, targeted treatments act with greater precision. They interfere with molecular signals that cancer cells rely on, limiting collateral damage to healthy tissue. In simple terms, if the tumor has a mutation in gene X and there is a treatment that targets cells with mutations in gene X, then we consider that treatment for the patient.

There are many (over one hundred as of this writing) FDA-approved targeted therapies available in various cancer types. This branch of oncology is expanding at an exponential pace, but below are several examples that are frequently used in practice today.

PARP Inhibitors for BRCA-Related and HRD-Positive Tumors

Some cancers, especially those linked to inherited BRCA1 or BRCA2 mutations, have a defect in DNA repair. But as we discussed in Chapter 5, **BRCA1 and BRCA2 are only two members of a larger family of homologous recombination repair genes**. Other genes in this pathway include **PALB2, RAD51C, RAD51D, BRIP1, BARD1, ATM, and CHEK2**, among others. When this pathway breaks down, the tumor is described as **homologous recombination deficient, or HRD**. PARP inhibitors take advantage of that weakness, regardless of which gene caused it, although BRCA-associated tumors still have the strongest and best-studied responses. Olaparib (Lynparza), rucaparib (Rubraca), and niraparib (Zejula) are oral drugs that block the enzyme poly (ADP-ribose) polymerase (PARP), preventing cancer cells from repairing their damaged DNA.

How This Works: The Concept of Synthetic Lethality

PARP inhibitors exploit a principle called synthetic lethality. The term sounds complicated, but the concept is elegant. *Synthetic* means artificially created, and *lethality* means death, so we're creating a deadly situation that wouldn't exist naturally.

To understand the concept, you need to know that your cells have multiple backup systems for repairing DNA damage. Think of them as different repair crews that fix different types of problems. The PARP enzyme handles small, single-stranded DNA breaks. The homologous recombination pathway (the HRD genes, including BRCA) handles large, double-stranded DNA breaks. In healthy cells, if one repair crew is unavailable, the other can compensate.

If you knock out just the PARP enzyme in normal cells, the cells can survive because the homologous recombination pathway can pick up the slack. If you knock out just the HRD pathway (like in BRCA-mutated cells), the cells can still survive by relying more heavily on the PARP pathway. But if you knock out *both* systems simultaneously, which is what happens when you give a PARP inhibitor to a tumor that already has HRD, the cancer cells have no way to repair their DNA damage. The combination is lethal, even though losing either system alone would not be.

This is why PARP inhibitors are so precisely targeted. They're relatively harmless to your normal cells (which have functional HRD and PARP systems), but deadly to tumor cells with HRD deficiency. The synthetic lethality strategy creates a therapeutic window where we can kill cancer cells without causing the widespread collateral damage typical of traditional chemotherapy. It's like a double strike effect: just like a batter who can't hit the fastball or the curveball will strike out, cancer cells that can't repair DNA damage through either pathway will die.

Who Benefits

PARP inhibitors have been especially effective in ovarian and breast cancers, among others. They are now often used as maintenance therapy to extend remission after chemotherapy or as treatment in advanced disease.

We use tumor and DNA testing to identify the patients most likely to benefit. In general, PARP inhibitors work best when the cancer has a weakness in one of its DNA repair systems. That weakness may be caused by:

- **An inherited BRCA1 or BRCA2 mutation**, found on germline testing
- **A BRCA1 or BRCA2 mutation found only in the tumor**, found on somatic tumor testing

- **HRD-positive status**, which means the tumor shows signs of a broader breakdown in the homologous recombination repair pathway, often involving genes beyond BRCA

This is a good example of precision medicine. Testing helps identify a weakness in the tumor, and PARP inhibitors are designed to take advantage of it. While BRCA-related cancers remain the best-known example, we now know that some tumors with broader HRD can also respond very well. That means these drugs may help more patients than we first thought when PARP inhibitors were used mainly for BRCA mutation carriers.

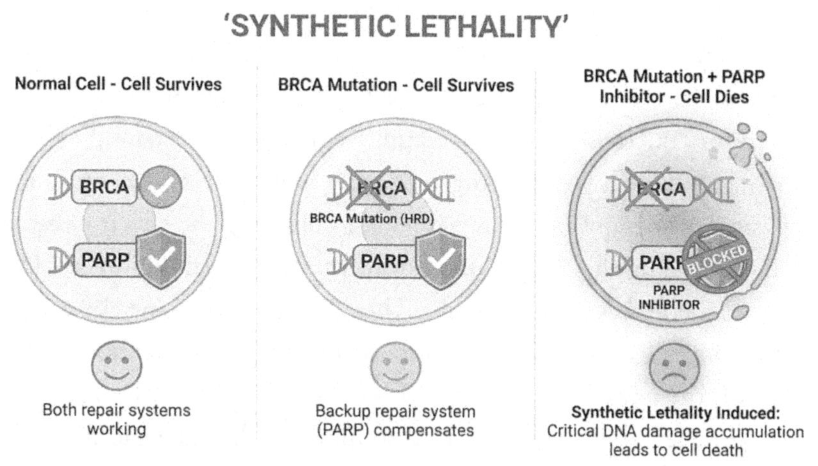

WORKBOOK CHECKPOINT: If you're receiving PARP inhibitors or other targeted therapy, complete page 7/3, **Section A: If I'm On Targeted Therapy.** Write down your specific target (BRCA/HRD, CDK4/6, HER2, etc.) and what to watch for.

CDK4/6 Inhibitors

For some women with ER-positive, HER2-negative breast cancer, CDK4/6 inhibitors, such as palbociclib (Ibrance), ribociclib (Kisqali), and abemaciclib (Verzenio), have become standard. These oral medications are created to block cancer cell growth by inhibiting the CDK4/6 protein from doing its job by interfering with the estrogen pathway. They are most commonly used in ER+ breast cancer in conjunction with anti-estrogen therapy, such as an aromatase inhibitor, like anastrozole (Arimidex), letrozole (Femara), or exemestane (Aromasin). They are also often combined with other anti-estrogen therapies, such as tamoxifen and fulvestrant (Faslodex).

CDK4/6 inhibitors greatly improve patient tumor response rates to hormone therapies by acting as a second brake in an ER+ breast cancer cell. One analogy to explain this is like a runaway train. The train represents estrogen receptor-positive (ER+) breast cancer cells, which are fueled by estrogen. Without intervention, the train keeps accelerating, representing the continued growth of these cancer cells. Anti-estrogen therapy is like the brakes on the train. Anti-estrogen therapy works by reducing or blocking the effects of estrogen, which in turn inhibits the growth of the cells. CDK4/6 inhibitors are like the next-level method to stop the train. These work by blocking the activity of enzymes that are critical for the cell to divide and survive. This action is like cutting off the power to the engine of the train. Therefore, the anti-estrogen therapy, like letrozole, and the CDK4/6 inhibitor, like abemaciclib, work in tandem to inhibit the cancer cells. Together, these treatments ensure that even if some cancer cells find a way to grow despite reduced estrogen, their ability to divide and proliferate is blocked. It's like ensuring that a train, once slowed down by the brakes, can't restart because its engine is disabled.

When combined with anti-estrogen therapy, CDK4/6 inhibitors can keep cancer in check for far longer than hormonal therapy alone. Increasingly, they are being used earlier in treatment, even after surgery, to reduce the risk of recurrence.

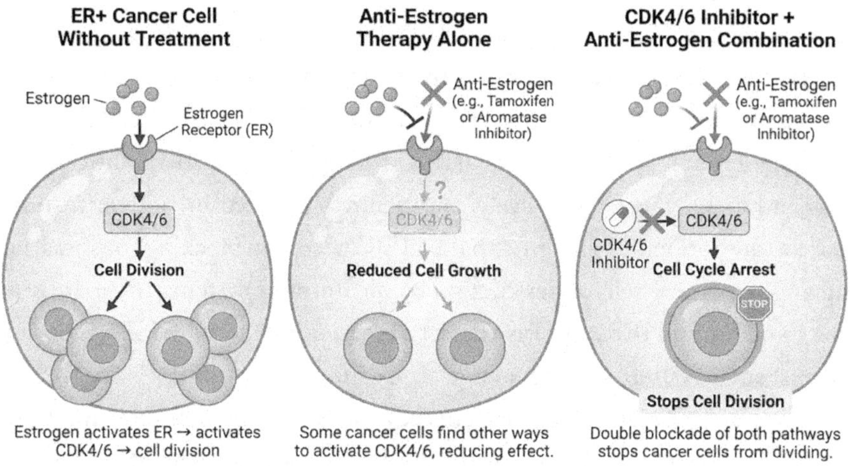

Patient Spotlight: Jane

Jane was a postmenopausal woman with stage II, ER-positive, HER2-negative breast cancer. After her lumpectomy and sentinel lymph node biopsy, her Oncotype score came back high, showing that her risk of recurrence was significant enough to warrant chemotherapy. She then completed radiation and began an aromatase inhibitor. Because her cancer also had higher-risk features, her doctors offered her a CDK4/6 inhibitor to add another layer of protection. Jane was hesitant to take yet another medication, but she ultimately decided to move forward because she wanted to do everything possible to reduce the chance of the cancer returning.

Anti-Angiogenic Therapy: Bevacizumab

One of the earliest targeted treatments in ovarian cancer was the use of bevacizumab (Avastin). This drug works by blocking a protein called VEGF, which stimulates new blood vessel growth. Tumors rely on these new blood vessels to bring in oxygen and nutrients. By shutting down this process, bevacizumab essentially starves the cancer and slows its growth. In ovarian cancer, it is sometimes given with chemotherapy in advanced cases, or continued as maintenance therapy afterward, or even in the setting of recurrent disease.

HER2-Targeted Therapy

In breast cancer, the development of HER2-targeted therapy changed outcomes dramatically. HER2 is a protein on the surface of some cancer cells that acts like an antenna, receiving signals that tell the cell to grow. In HER2-positive cancers, there are too many copies of this protein, which can drive the cancer to grow and spread more aggressively. Trastuzumab (Herceptin) and pertuzumab (Perjeta) are antibodies that bind to the HER2 receptor, blocking the signal and flagging the cancer cell for destruction by the immune system. These drugs are now standard for HER2-positive breast cancer, as well as other HER2-positive cancers, such as uterine, lung, and gastric cancers.

Newer HER2-directed treatments have become even more effective. Drugs such as ado-trastuzumab emtansine (Kadcyla) and trastuzumab deruxtecan (Enhertu) build on the success of trastuzumab by using the HER2 antibody as a delivery system for chemotherapy. For many patients, these therapies have turned what was once one of the most aggressive forms of breast cancer into a much more treatable disease. We will review these in the next section.

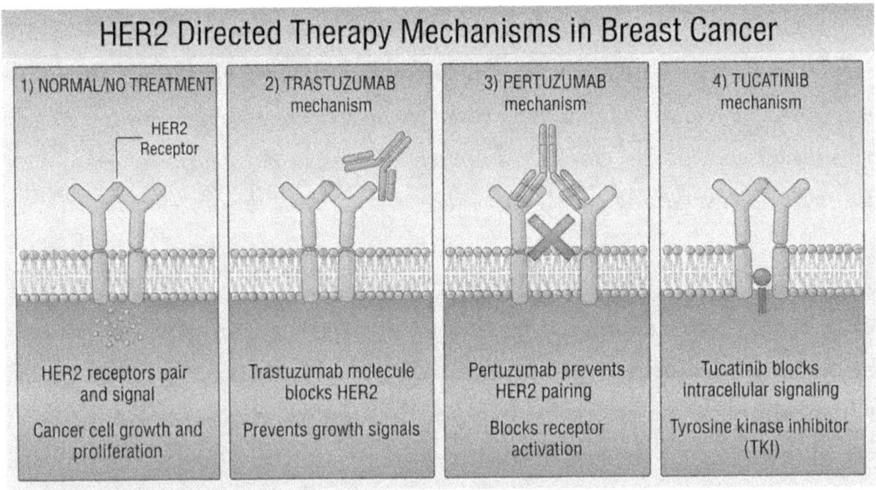

Antibody–Drug Conjugates (ADCs): The Next Generation

A newer and rapidly expanding category of targeted therapies is called antibody–drug conjugates (ADCs). These represent some of the most exciting advances in cancer treatment that I have seen in my career. ADCs are like precision-guided missiles that can seek out cancer cells and deliver a powerful chemotherapy payload directly inside them.

How ADCs Work

ADCs combine three key components: an antibody that acts like a GPS system to find specific proteins on cancer cells, a potent chemotherapy drug (often much stronger than traditional chemo), and a special linker that holds them together until the right moment. The antibody part binds to a specific target on the cancer cell surface (such as the HER2 receptor). Once attached, the entire ADC gets pulled inside the cell, where the linker breaks apart and releases the chemotherapy directly into the cancer cell. This approach allows us to use much more powerful drugs than we could give systemically, while limiting damage to healthy cells.

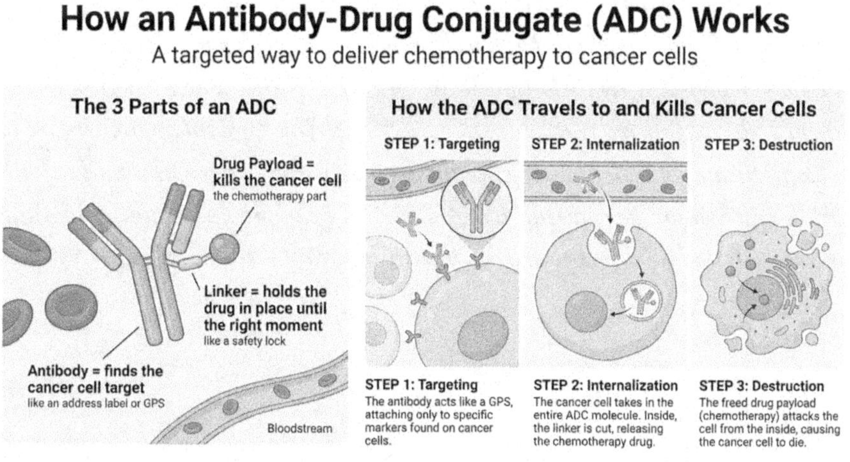

ADCs in Clinical Practice

Several ADCs have transformed treatment for patients whose cancers have become resistant to other therapies. Trastuzumab deruxtecan (Enhertu) has shown remarkable results not only in HER2-positive breast and gastric cancers but also in HER2-low breast cancers, a group for which we previously had few targeted options. This drug has been so effective that it has changed how we think about HER2 as a target.

Some other examples of ADCs include:

- Sacituzumab govitecan (Trodelvy) targets a protein called Trop-2, which is found on many breast cancer cells. For women with metastatic triple-negative breast cancer, this ADC has provided new hope when other treatments have stopped working.
- Mirvetuximab soravtansine (Elahere) targets folate receptor alpha and has been approved for platinum-resistant ovarian cancer, offering a targeted therapy specifically for this challenging group of patients.

Patient Spotlight: Anna

Recall Anna? She is the forty-eight-year-old attorney with metastatic HER2-positive breast cancer. She first responded very well to chemotherapy plus anti-HER2 antibodies and even achieved a remission based on her PET scans. When her cancer later returned, she was offered trastuzumab deruxtecan. This targeted approach gave her renewed disease control, allowing her to continue working part-time and enjoying her role as a mentor. For patients like Anna, ADCs can provide meaningful disease control with a more targeted approach than traditional chemotherapy.

WORKBOOK CHECKPOINT: If you're receiving an ADC like Anna, turn to workbook page 7/4, **My ADC Guide**, to document your specific GPS target and the unique side effects to watch for. ADCs are precision treatments, and understanding yours will help you partner effectively with your medical team.

The Promise and Challenges

What makes ADCs so exciting is their potential to deliver powerful treatment directly to cancer cells while sparing healthy tissues compared with traditional chemotherapy. However, they can still cause side effects. Unlike traditional chemotherapy, where we expect certain predictable side effects, ADCs can cause toxicity through some unexpected pathways. Sometimes the drug gets released from the antibody before it reaches the cancer cell, like a package coming unwrapped during delivery. When this happens, the powerful chemotherapy payload can affect healthy cells it was never meant to target.

Other times, normal cells in your body can mistakenly pick up the ADC even though they do not have the target protein we are trying to hit. For example, immune cells called macrophages have receptors that can grab onto antibodies, including ADCs. This is why we sometimes see lung problems with trastuzumab deruxtecan because the immune cells in the lung can take up the drug even though the lung tissue itself does not have the HER2 protein. Once inside these cells, the chemotherapy gets released and can cause inflammation of the lungs (pneumon*itis*). ADCs can likewise cause inflammation in other organs such as the thyroid (thyroid*itis*), the colon (col*itis*), or the liver (hepat*itis*). These inflammatory reactions often reverse when the ADC is stopped or treated with steroids, but in some instances, they can be longer-lasting.

The bystander effect is another factor. When an ADC delivers its payload to a cancer cell, some of that drug can leak out and affect nearby cells that happen to be in the neighborhood. If the nearby cells are healthy cells, then the result is a toxicity or a side effect. But in some cases, if the nearby cells are cancer, then it is a beneficial added benefit. Interestingly, this type of side effect mostly has to do with how the ADC is built, particularly the linker that holds the antibody and chemotherapy together. ADCs with unstable linkers tend to *leak* their chemotherapy payload and cause more problems throughout the body.

The good news is that researchers are getting better at designing ADCs with more stable linkers and smarter delivery systems. The number of ADCs currently in development is astounding. We are also learning to use them earlier in patient treatment regimens and in combination with other therapies, such as immunotherapy. I am very encouraged by how fast things are developing in this field, and I believe ADCs will play a very significant role in cancer treatments in the future.

Looking Ahead

Systemic therapy has expanded far beyond traditional chemotherapy, offering options that are more precise, more effective, and often more tolerable than in the past. Your oncologist will determine whether chemotherapy, immunotherapy, hormone therapy, targeted therapy, antibody-drug conjugates, or a combination of these approaches is right for you. That decision is shaped by many factors, including the type and stage of cancer, the presence of specific proteins or genetic mutations in the tumor, and your overall health and treatment goals.

The era of personalized medicine means that treatment plans are no longer one-size-fits-all. Instead, they are designed to target your cancer's unique profile while minimizing unnecessary toxicity. This individualized approach aims not only to control or cure the disease but also to preserve your quality of life throughout treatment and beyond.

When You Face Treatment Choices

Sometimes your oncologist will present more than one reasonable treatment option, each with different risks, benefits, and trade-offs. You will likely find yourself weighing options such as choosing between chemotherapy regimens, deciding whether to add a targeted therapy, or considering clinical trial enrollment. This chapter is dense, and you have been given a lot to absorb about systemic therapy. The worksheets in this chapter are meant to help you organize what you have learned, add your own thoughts and questions, and clarify what matters most to you. My goal is to help you be prepared for shared decision-making conversations with your medical team and get your best possible cancer outcome.

WORKBOOK CHECKPOINT: I want to review the worksheets included with this chapter since there are several of them. Please note that not all worksheets will be applicable to everyone. For example, some of you will have chemotherapy, some will have hormone therapy, and some will have both. Just skip the ones that do not apply to you.

- **My Systemic Therapy Overview** Chapter 7, page 1 (everyone)
- **Understanding My Hormone Therapy** Chapter 7, page 2
- **Targeted Therapy and Immunotherapy Tracker** Chapter 7, page 3
- **My ADC Guide** Chapter 7, page 4
- **Questions to Ask My Medical Oncologist** Chapter 7, page 5 (everyone)
- **Treatment Decision Worksheet** Chapter 7, page 6 (everyone)

- **My Systemic Therapy Timeline** Chapter 7, page 7 (everyone)
- Please update your worksheet from Chapter 3, page 5: **My Medical Oncology Team Contact Sheet** with any new numbers (everyone)
- Also, update any new dates and schedules in your **Cancer Journey Planner** (everyone)

Remember: You don't have to understand everything perfectly right now. These workbook pages are tools to help you organize information, ask better questions, and feel more in control as you move forward. Return to them as often as you need.

Chapter 8

Radiation Made Clear: What It Does and What You Can Expect

Introduction to Radiation Therapy

Radiation therapy is one of the three main tools doctors use to treat cancer, alongside surgery and systemic treatments like chemotherapy or hormone therapy. At its core, radiation uses invisible beams of high-energy particles to damage the DNA inside cancer cells so they can no longer grow or divide. Unlike chemotherapy, which travels throughout the body, radiation is what we call a *local therapy* because it treats a specific part of the body while leaving the rest untouched.

Many women feel unsettled when they first hear the word *radiation.* It may call up images of nuclear disasters or science-fiction movies. The reality in cancer care is very different. Modern radiation therapy is carefully designed, precisely targeted, and safer than ever before. Think of it as a spotlight rather than a floodlight, which shines exactly where it's needed.

Radiation has been used to treat cancer for more than a century, but the way we deliver it has changed dramatically. What began as a crude, one-size-fits-all approach has become a highly sophisticated therapy guided by advanced imaging, computer planning, and specialized machines that can bend and shape beams to match the exact outline of a tumor.

WORKBOOK CHECKPOINT: Before you begin radiation therapy, take a moment to update your **My Healthcare Providers** (page 3/5) with your radiation oncology team information. Having all your providers in one central document ensures seamless communication across your entire care team.

How Radiation Works

Radiation therapy works by damaging the DNA inside cells. DNA, or deoxyribonucleic acid, is the instruction manual that tells every cell in your body how to grow, divide, and function. When radiation strikes, it creates tiny breaks in the DNA strands. A healthy cell has repair mechanisms that can often fix this damage. A cancer cell, however, usually has faulty repair pathways; the DNA damage overwhelms it, leading to cell death or permanent loss of the ability to divide.

There are two main ways radiation injures cells. The first is *direct damage*, when the energy from radiation directly breaks the DNA strands. The second is *indirect damage*, when radiation interacts with water molecules inside the cell and produces highly reactive particles known as *free radicals*. These free radicals then damage the DNA further. Together, these effects tip the balance against cancer cells, which are already genetically unstable.

Importantly, radiation therapy is not felt while it is being delivered. Patients do not feel heat, burning, or pain during treatment; the energy passes invisibly and silently into the body. The effects unfold over time as cancer cells attempt and fail to repair their damaged DNA.

Types of Radiation Therapy

There is no single type of radiation therapy. Over the past decades, technology has advanced so much that we can now shape, guide, and deliver radiation in highly individualized ways. Broadly speaking, radiation is given in three forms: external beam radiation, internal radiation, and systemic radiation.

External Beam Radiation Therapy (EBRT)

This is the most common form of radiation. A machine called a linear accelerator generates beams of high-energy X-rays or particles that are directed from outside the body toward the tumor. The patient lies on a treatment table while the machine rotates around them, delivering radiation from different angles to focus on the cancer and spare as much normal tissue as possible.

Within external beam radiation, there are several specialized approaches:

- **Three-Dimensional Conformal Radiation Therapy (3D-CRT):** uses imaging to shape beams to the exact dimensions of the tumor.
- **Intensity-Modulated Radiation Therapy (IMRT):** adjusts the strength, or intensity, of beams across different areas, allowing for more precise control and reduced side effects.
- **Image-Guided Radiation Therapy (IGRT) and Volumetric Modulated Arc Therapy (VMAT):** often used together and are advanced technologies. IGRT uses frequent imaging during treatment to ensure accuracy, especially when tumors may move with breathing or digestion. And VMAT is the improved and faster form of IMRT, where the machine rotates around the patient and delivers radiation in only one to two minutes.
- **Stereotactic Radiosurgery (SRS) and Stereotactic Body Radiotherapy (SBRT):** deliver very high doses in one to five sessions with pinpoint accuracy. SRS is often used for brain tumors and can also be used for small tumors in the lung, liver, or spine.

- **Proton Beam Therapy:** instead of X-rays, protons (positively charged particles) are used. Protons release most of their energy directly at the tumor, then stop, which means less radiation is delivered to tissues beyond the target. This can be especially helpful in children or when tumors are near sensitive organs.
- **Carbon Ion Therapy:** an emerging technology, not yet widely available in the United States, that uses heavier particles than protons. Carbon ions deliver more energy within the tumor and have greater biological effectiveness, making them promising for cancers that resist conventional radiation.

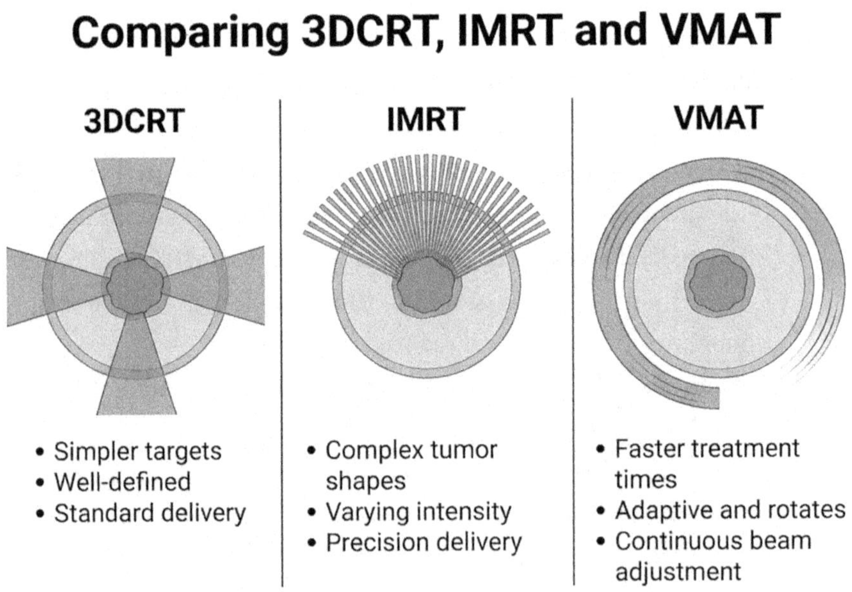

Internal Radiation Therapy (Brachytherapy)

In some cases, the most effective way to deliver radiation is from inside the body. Brachytherapy involves placing radioactive material directly into or next to the tumor. Thin tubes, seeds, or ribbons containing the radioactive source are inserted for either a short period (temporary brachytherapy) or left in place permanently. This method is commonly used in gynecologic cancers such as cervical or endometrial cancer, as well as in prostate cancer.

Systemic Radiation Therapy

With systemic radiotherapy, radioactive substances are swallowed or injected into the bloodstream. They circulate throughout the body and target cancer cells wherever they are.

A classic example of this technique is the use of radioactive iodine (I-131) for thyroid cancer, where the thyroid cells absorb the radionucleotide specifically. Radium-223 is another well-established option. This molecule is drawn to bone and can reduce pain from prostate cancer that has spread to the skeleton.

The newest advances involve radiopharmaceuticals. These are radioactive particles linked to antibodies or small molecules designed to find cancer cells. Similar to how ADCs use antibodies or targeting molecules as GPS systems, radiopharmaceuticals attach radioactive particles to molecules that lock onto specific features on cancer cells. The antibody acts like a homing device. It guides the radioactive payload directly to the tumor while minimizing exposure to healthy tissue. This approach is sometimes called targeted radiotherapy or radioimmunotherapy. Lutetium-177 PSMA (prostate-specific membrane antigen) is one example. It delivers radiation directly to prostate cancer cells that express the PSMA protein.

This field is also expanding through the concept of theranostics, which pairs a diagnostic scan with a targeted treatment. First, you receive an injection of a diagnostic tracer, a small amount of radioactive material designed to light up on a special scan and show doctors exactly where your cancer cells are located. Once the precise locations are mapped out, you get a second injection containing a therapeutic agent, which uses the same targeting molecule but now carries a much higher dose of radiation. The treatment travels through your bloodstream, locks onto those same cancer spots, and destroys them. For example, gallium-68 PSMA (prostate-specific membrane antigen) PET scans can reveal prostate cancer deposits throughout the body, and then lutetium-177 PSMA can be used to treat those exact locations. This *search-and-destroy* approach personalizes radiation therapy to a specific cancer type.

Each of these methods of radiation delivery and use has its place. The choice depends on the location of the tumor, its size, the patient's overall health, and whether the goal is cure or symptom relief.

WORKBOOK CHECKPOINT: Now that you understand the different types of radiation therapy, turn to page 8/1, **My Radiation Therapy Overview**, in your Workbook. Fill in which type you'll be receiving, your treatment goal, and the key details about your schedule.

Indications for Radiation

Radiation therapy is not given in the same way for every cancer. Its role depends on the type of tumor, the stage, and whether the goal is cure or control. Doctors think of radiation in four main categories.

Adjuvant Radiation (After Surgery)

Radiation is often recommended after surgery to lower the risk of cancer returning in the same area. Even when a surgeon removes all visible disease, microscopic cancer cells can remain behind. Radiation is used to destroy these cells and secure the best chance for long-term control. This is especially common in breast cancer, where women who undergo a lumpectomy almost always receive adjuvant radiation.

Patient Spotlight: Jane

Jane was fifty-five when a mammogram revealed a Stage II breast cancer. After a lumpectomy and chemotherapy, her doctors recommended adjuvant radiation to the left breast. While the surgery had removed the tumor, the radiation provided a safety net against cells too small to see. This additional step reduced her risk of local recurrence and gave her confidence that she was doing everything possible to put cancer behind her.

Post-Mastectomy Radiation

Some women require radiation even after the entire breast has been removed. When tumors are large or lymph nodes are involved, radiation is used to treat the chest wall or regional lymph node areas. This added step provides an extra layer of protection against recurrence, particularly in aggressive breast cancers.

Neoadjuvant Radiation (Before Surgery)

In certain cancers, radiation is given before surgery to shrink a tumor and make it easier to remove. Rectal cancer is a classic example: a course of radiation can reduce the tumor size, improve the likelihood of a complete resection, and lessen the chance of recurrence.

Curative Radiation Alone (Definitive Radiation)

For some cancers, radiation itself can be the main treatment. Cervical cancer, prostate cancer, and certain head and neck cancers may be cured with radiation, sometimes combined with chemotherapy. In these situations, radiation takes the place of surgery.

Palliative Radiation (For Symptom Relief)

Radiation is also used when a cure is not possible, but relief is. A short course of treatment can ease pain from bone metastases, shrink a tumor pressing on an organ, or control bleeding. Even a single session can make a profound difference in quality of life.

Patient Spotlight: Anna

Anna, a forty-eight-year-old attorney, learned she had Stage IV breast cancer after suffering a painful rib fracture. Scans revealed that cancer had spread to her bones.

Her oncologist used palliative radiation to the ribs to relieve her pain and reduce the risk of further fractures. The treatment allowed her to continue working part-time and, more importantly, to keep mentoring young attorneys—something that brought her deep joy. In Anna's case, radiation was not about a cure but about regaining comfort and control in her daily life.

How Radiation Is Administered

Radiation treatment does not begin the moment a patient walks into the department. Careful planning is essential to make sure the beams reach the tumor with precision while protecting as much normal tissue as possible.

The process starts with a **simulation**, which is a planning session rather than a treatment. During this visit, patients are positioned exactly as they will be for every treatment that follows. Special molds, cushions, or masks may be made to keep the body still and in the same alignment each day. A CT scan is performed in this position; this imaging allows the radiation team to map the tumor and surrounding structures in three dimensions.

Once the images are obtained, the radiation oncologist, along with medical physicists and dosimetrists (specialists who calculate radiation dose), uses sophisticated computer programs to design the treatment plan. They decide the angles, strengths, and shapes of the beams to maximize tumor coverage and minimize radiation to normal tissues.

When treatment begins, it is usually delivered in small daily doses called **fractions**. Most patients come five days a week, with the full course lasting anywhere from one to seven weeks, depending on the cancer type and the treatment goal. Each session lasts only a few minutes, and the patient feels nothing as the radiation is delivered. The machine may move around the body, but it does not touch the patient, and the beams themselves are invisible.

Behind the scenes, the care team works in close coordination. The **radiation oncologist** oversees the entire process and monitors progress. **Radiation therapists** operate the machines and guide patients through their daily treatments. **Medical physicists** and **dosimetrists** ensure the accuracy and safety of every plan. **Nurses** provide education, symptom management, and emotional support throughout the process. Radiation therapy is a team effort; patients are never going through it alone.

Patient Spotlight: Lydia

Lydia was forty-five when she faced triple-negative breast cancer. After chemotherapy and a bilateral mastectomy, her doctors recommended post-mastectomy radiation to lower her risk of recurrence. She admitted she was terrified of the treatment, not because of side effects but because of the machine itself. The idea of lying flat, arms raised, with a massive machine circling her body triggered her claustrophobia.

During her simulation, the team walked her step-by-step through what would happen. They explained that the treatment would be brief, that she would not feel the beams, and that therapists would watch her closely on a camera and microphone the entire time. The first few sessions were difficult, but Lydia developed small mental strategies: controlled breathing, visualizing a safe place, and reminding herself that each minute on the table was another step toward long-term health. By the end of her course, she described the process as "Easier than I ever imagined," not because it was pleasant but because she learned how to prepare herself emotionally and trusted her team.

WORKBOOK CHECKPOINT: Your simulation appointment is a crucial planning session. Before you go, review workbook page 8/2, **My Simulation & Planning Appointment**. After the simulation, fill in the details about your immobilization device, tattoo markings, and timeline until your first treatment. Don't forget to mark important radiation-related appointments in your Planner in the Monthly pages as well.

Side Effects and What to Expect

Radiation is powerful, but it is also precise. The goal is always to treat the cancer while sparing as much healthy tissue as possible. Even with the best planning, however, radiation can cause side effects. These vary depending on the part of the body being treated, the dose, and the length of therapy.

The most common side effect across all types of radiation is **fatigue**. This is not the kind of tiredness that goes away with a good night's sleep. It can feel more like a deep heaviness, as if the body is spending extra energy on healing that you cannot see. Patients often describe it as "slowing down a gear."

Another common issue is a **skin change** in the treated area. This may look like a sunburn—redness, dryness, or mild peeling. In most cases, the skin heals fully, but gentle care is important. Radiation teams provide specific instructions on moisturizers, clothing, and avoiding harsh soaps or perfumes on the affected skin.

Side effects can also be **site-specific**. For example, radiation to the head and neck can cause dry mouth or difficulty swallowing. Radiation to the pelvis may affect the bladder or bowels. Breast or chest wall radiation can cause tightness or swelling in the treated area. Long-term complications are much less common than they once were, but doctors always discuss them as part of the planning process so that patients can make informed choices.

Patient Spotlight: Lydia

For Lydia, fatigue was the most noticeable side effect. She described it as a wave that rolled in late in the afternoon, making her want to crawl into bed earlier than usual. The skin over her chest also grew pink and tender as the weeks went by, though it never became painful. What surprised her most was how manageable these effects were once she knew what to expect. By pacing her day, resting when her body signaled the need, and keeping up with the skin care routine provided by her radiation nurses, Lydia completed her full course of treatment without interruption. She later told me that the anticipation was far worse than the reality; once she was in the rhythm, the treatments became part of her routine, not the center of her life.

WORKBOOK CHECKPOINT: Please refer to page 8/3, **Questions to Ask My Radiation Oncologist** and page 8/4, **What to Expect—Radiation Side Effects Guide**, which explains what to expect, and use your Cancer Journey Planner to track how you're feeling day-by-day. Document your energy levels, skin condition, and any new symptoms in real time.

Summary

Radiation therapy is one of the central tools in cancer care. It can be given with the intent to cure, to lower the chance of recurrence, or to relieve symptoms when a cure is not possible. Today's radiation is far more precise than in the past; beams are shaped to match the tumor, treatment is guided by advanced imaging, and doses are carefully calculated by a team of specialists. While side effects, such as fatigue and skin irritation, are common, most are temporary and manageable with good preparation and support. Radiation is not something to fear—it is a carefully controlled treatment designed to target cancer while protecting the rest of the body.

Advances and Future Directions

Radiation therapy has changed more in the last few decades than in the entire century before it, and progress continues at a rapid pace. Proton therapy is becoming more widely available, especially for children and tumors located near sensitive organs. Carbon ion therapy, used in a few centers worldwide, delivers even greater biological effectiveness and may help cancers that resist other treatments.

The theranostic approach we discussed earlier is expanding rapidly. Doctors use one scan to find your cancer and another treatment to target it. Right now, it's mainly used for prostate cancer, but researchers are testing it for breast cancer, lung cancer, and other types. The goal is to figure out which patients will benefit most. They also want to fine-tune the doses based on what each person's cancer looks like. As scientists discover more molecular targets on cancer cells, this personalized *search-and-destroy* strategy will become an option for more and more people.

Researchers are also studying how radiation can be combined with immunotherapy. In some cases, radiation to one tumor can actually wake up your immune system. It gets your immune system to attack cancer elsewhere in your body. This phenomenon is called the abscopal effect. Doctors are working hard to understand how to make this happen more reliably (Skaznik-Wikiel et al. 2018).

The good news is that radiation therapy has evolved significantly. Treatments are more precise. Side effects are better managed. New approaches like proton therapy and theranostics are expanding treatment options.

Part III

Receiving Treatment

Chapter 9

The Pre-Treatment Playbook: What to Do Before Day One

Welcome to Chapter 9, where we focus on what you need to do before starting chemotherapy and preparations to consider before each treatment cycle. This chapter is designed to help you understand the practical aspects of preparation and what to expect from the treatment process. We'll explore different aspects of treatment preparation, and medical devices like a mediport, techniques like cold capping, and how to communicate effectively with your healthcare team about care preferences.

In addition, I will give you some suggestions on how to organize your personal life to ease the impact of chemotherapy. This includes arranging transportation, meal preparation, and managing your work schedule, so you have the support you need during a challenging time in your life.

By the end of this chapter, I hope you will have a clear understanding of how to prepare for chemotherapy logistically and mentally. The goal is to reduce stress through preparation and make your treatment as smooth and manageable as possible.

WORKBOOK CHECKPOINT: Before diving into the details, turn to page 9/1, **My Pre-Treatment Preparation Checklist,** in your workbook. This master checklist will serve as your roadmap throughout this chapter. As you read each section, you can check off the corresponding items on page 9/1 to ensure nothing falls through the cracks. Having one central checklist reduces anxiety and gives you a clear sense of progress as you prepare for day one.

Mediport Placement and Usage

For many patients, the idea of starting chemotherapy is made even more stressful by the thought of repeated IV sticks. A mediport, sometimes called a port-a-cath, is a small device placed under the skin, usually in the upper chest, that becomes your reliable *access site* for treatment. Instead of searching for a vein each time, your care team can safely and comfortably deliver chemotherapy directly into the bloodstream through this port.

The placement itself is a minor surgical procedure. You'll be given local anesthesia, sometimes with light sedation, so you're relaxed and comfortable. The surgeon makes a small incision in the chest to tuck the port under the skin, and another tiny opening near the collarbone or neck where the catheter is guided into a large vein that leads to the heart (the superior vena cava). Once it's in place, it's invisible under clothing but easy for your team to access.

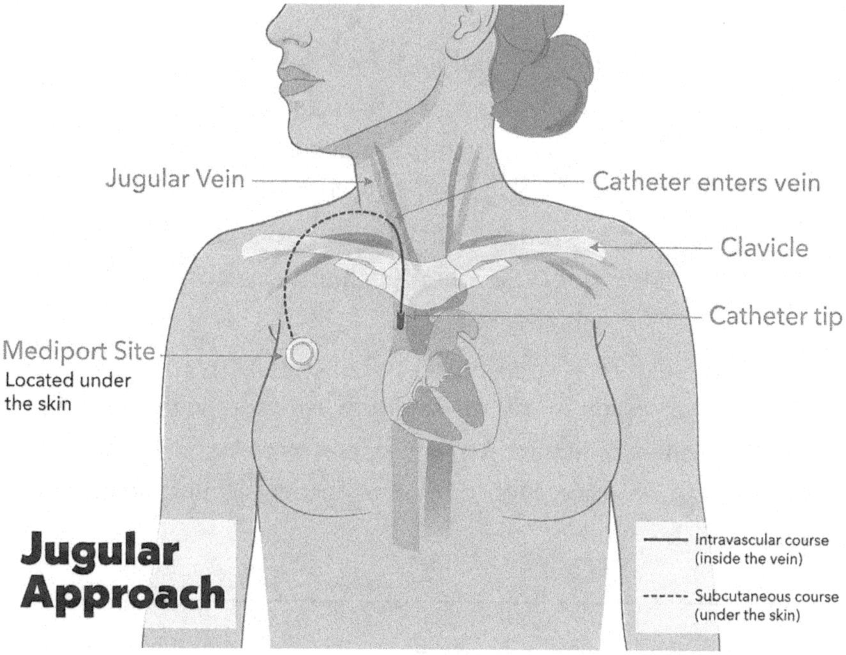

Patient Spotlight: Anna

I recall that initially, Anna was reluctant to have a mediport placed. She felt like "it was too many things to do and think about" in the beginning. Understanding her position, we agreed to revisit the discussion after she had a few treatments under her belt. After her third infusion through a vein in her arm, she left with large bruises and worried her veins wouldn't hold up. Before her next cycle, she admitted, "I'm more scared of the IV than the chemo itself at this point, and I am worried that they won't be able to get my IV placed next time." We then spent some time reviewing what the port was, how it worked, and how it would be inserted under local anesthesia. Once her port was placed, she actually felt a lot of relief. Each infusion was straightforward: no more multiple sticks, no more arm bruising, and her veins were preserved for the future. She told me the port gave her back some sense of control, and it was one less thing to worry about at each visit.

PRO TIP: Ask your oncologist for a prescription for topical lidocaine cream (one common brand is EMLA). About an hour before your appointment, place a pea-sized amount over the port site and cover it with plastic wrap. By the time your nurse is ready to access the port, the skin will be numb, making needle placement far more comfortable.

When your session is finished, the nurse removes the needle and places a small Band-Aid over the site. You can shower, exercise, and go about daily life with the port in place. Over time, many patients almost forget it's there until it's needed.

WORKBOOK CHECKPOINT: If you're having a mediport placed, turn to page 9/2, **My Mediport Information Card**, in your workbook. Fill in the details after your placement procedure—date, location, type, and care instructions. This card becomes your quick reference for every infusion appointment and for any emergency situation. Keep a photo of the completed card on your phone so you always have the information handy. Don't forget the Pro Tip: request a prescription for topical lidocaine cream.

Cold Capping

One of the hardest side effects of chemotherapy is hair loss. For many women, hair is tied not only to appearance but also to identity. Losing it can feel like losing a part of yourself. Some women fear that being bald will make their cancer visible to the world, when they would rather keep that part of their life private. Others want to hide treatment from coworkers to avoid being treated differently at work. Parents often worry about how hair loss will affect their young children, who may not fully understand what is happening.

At the same time, some women choose not to pursue cold capping at all. For them, shaving their head and embracing baldness feels freeing. It can be a powerful statement of strength, a way of saying, "I will not hide from this." Both choices are valid. Cold capping is not about what you should do, but about what may help you feel most comfortable and authentic during treatment.

Cold capping, also called scalp cooling, is a technique designed to help preserve hair during chemotherapy. The process involves wearing a specially designed cap chilled to very low temperatures before, during, and after your infusion. The cold constricts blood vessels in the scalp, limiting the amount of chemotherapy that reaches the hair follicles. With less drug exposure, there is a greater chance that the follicles will survive, and the hair will stay intact.

Cold capping is not a guarantee. Some chemotherapy drugs, such as doxorubicin or full-dose docetaxel, cause hair loss even with scalp cooling. The treatment can also be physically uncomfortable. The frozen cap must stay in place for hours, and some patients experience headaches or scalp pain. The process extends the time you will spend in the infusion center, since the cap needs to be worn before and after chemotherapy.

There are ways to make cold capping easier to tolerate. Practicing with the cap ahead of time by putting it on and off yourself can reduce anxiety about the fit. Taking Tylenol before treatment can help with headaches, and if needed, your team may offer antianxiety medication, such as lorazepam, to help you stay comfortable.

Insurance coverage has improved in recent years. Medicare began covering scalp cooling in 2022, and most private insurance companies now cover cold capping as well, although prior authorization from your doctor's office is often still required.

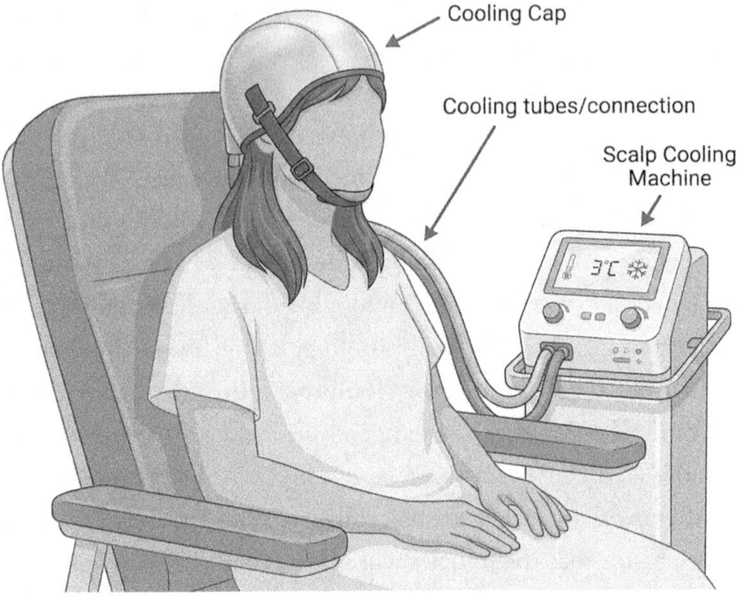

Patient Spotlight: Laura

Laura was deeply reluctant to start chemotherapy, and she had multiple concerns. It turns out that one of them was losing her hair. When I asked her to list the reasons, she was hesitant about the treatment. She paused, then admitted how unhappy she was at the thought of being bald. For her, hair loss symbolized the loss of normalcy and control. Together, we reviewed her treatment plan and discussed how cold capping could help. Since scalp cooling must begin with the very first chemotherapy infusion, we adjusted her schedule so that her chemotherapy treatment, paclitaxel, could be given weekly at a lower dose rather than every three weeks. This allowed the cold cap to be more effective. Laura decided to go forward with treatment, encouraged by the possibility of preserving her hair. It gave her a sense that she was not only fighting her cancer but also protecting a part of her identity.

WORKBOOK CHECKPOINT: If you're considering cold capping, turn to page 9/3, **Cold Capping Decision and Preparation Guide** in your workbook. This page will help you think through whether cold capping is right for you, understand the financial and physical commitments, and organize the logistics. Remember: cold capping must begin with your very first chemotherapy infusion, so this decision needs to be made before treatment starts. If you're uncertain, discuss it with your oncologist at your next appointment—don't wait until the last minute.

Health Care Proxy (HCP)

Before beginning chemotherapy or any major medical treatment, it is essential to confirm who will make decisions for you if you are unable to do so yourself. This person is called your health care proxy (HCP). Choosing and documenting an HCP may feel uncomfortable, but it is one of the most empowering steps you can take. It ensures that your wishes are respected, even in situations where you cannot speak for yourself.

An HCP is usually a trusted family member or close friend who understands your values and will advocate for you. Having these conversations early allows your medical team to know who should be contacted if a critical decision arises. Once completed, the form should be filed with your oncology team, included in your cancer binder, and shared with the person you've chosen so they are prepared.

Another important role of the HCP is serving as a safeguard for your privacy. Medical offices are only permitted to release information to the person you've designated, which means your health details are filtered through someone you trust. This protects you from having sensitive information shared too widely and helps manage communication with extended family and friends.

Most hospitals, cancer centers, and state health websites provide downloadable health care proxy forms. These forms are often state-specific, and your oncology office can guide you through the paperwork. In some states, the document may need to be witnessed or notarized, so ask your care team about the rules where you live.

WORKBOOK CHECKPOINT: Once you've completed your Healthcare Proxy form, check it off on page 9/1, **My Pre-Treatment Preparation Checklist**. Make sure copies are filed with your oncology team, included in your Cancer Journey Binder, and given to the person you've designated. This is one of those tasks that feels uncomfortable but provides enormous peace of mind once it's done.

Fertility Preservation

As discussed in Chapter 3, if you are of childbearing age and have not yet addressed fertility preservation, this is your last checkpoint before starting chemotherapy. Once treatment begins, the window for preserving eggs or embryos closes. If this is something you want to explore, speak with your oncologist **immediately** about delaying treatment by ten to fourteen days to pursue fertility preservation. Please refer back to Chapter 3 for a detailed discussion of your options, or ask your care team for an urgent referral to a reproductive endocrinologist. **Don't let this decision be made by default.** The decision should be made consciously with full information and support.

Preparing Your Schedule and Household

Chemotherapy does not just affect your body; it reshapes your daily rhythm. The best way to navigate this shift is by planning ahead, so your energy is spent on recovery rather than scrambling to keep life on track.

Start with transportation. If you normally drive yourself or your children, arrange for backup during the days right after treatment. Even if you feel well enough to get behind the wheel, fatigue, nausea, or medications can make driving unsafe. Knowing you have a plan takes away the last-minute stress of asking for help.

Meals are another area where preparation pays off. Stock your freezer with easy, nourishing options or set up a meal delivery schedule with friends or family. This prevents you from relying on takeout when your appetite is unpredictable or when grocery shopping feels overwhelming. Many patients often resist having others help them because they want to maintain their regular routine. But accepting help, even when you feel you could manage on your own, is not a sign of weakness. Letting others help you is a way of protecting your strength for the moments you truly need it, since fatigue, nausea, and other symptoms can catch you off guard.

Your work schedule also deserves attention. Plan to take two to three days off after your first cycle to see how your body responds. Some people bounce back quickly, while others need more recovery time. For later cycles, you may be able to adjust your routine, but avoid overextending yourself. Flexibility is key, since side effects can vary from one infusion to the next.

Finally, focus on the basics of self-care that directly support recovery. Stay well hydrated, eat small, frequent meals, and alternate activity with rest. Keep track of bowel movements, since both constipation and diarrhea are common during treatment and can usually be managed if caught early. Use your planner to record your symptoms with details, so your medical team can step in quickly if problems arise.

By being prepared, you are setting up a safety net in case you are not feeling well or are too fatigued to carry on your regular responsibilities. The more you set up ahead of time, the less stress you will feel during and after your treatments.

Patient Spotlight: Anna

Recall Anna, who is a busy attorney. At the beginning of her treatment, she insisted she could manage chemotherapy without disrupting her schedule. She planned court appearances and client meetings right after her first infusion, determined not to let cancer slow her down. Within two days, she was completely exhausted, struggling with nausea, and frustrated that she could not meet her own expectations. After that experience, we sat down and made a different plan. She arranged for colleagues to cover her early court dates, accepted meal help from friends, and built in recovery days after each treatment. Anna admits that letting go of control is difficult, but she has learned that protecting her strength allows her to be more present for her clients in the long run and gives her the reserves she needs to get through treatment.

WORKBOOK CHECKPOINT: Return to page 9/1, **My Pre-Treatment Preparation Checklist**, and review the Household and Logistics section. Check off the items you've already arranged—transportation, meals, work schedule, childcare—and identify what still needs attention. Don't try to do everything yourself. Accepting help now, even when you feel capable, preserves your strength for the moments when you truly need it. Remember Anna's lesson: protecting your energy allows you to show up more fully for what matters most.

Reviewing Treatment Information

Before starting chemotherapy, it is important to review and understand the treatment plan your oncology team has prepared for you. Knowing what to expect will help reduce anxiety and give you more confidence as you begin.

Go over the details of your chemotherapy drugs, how they are given, and what side effects are most likely. Depending on your specific treatment, your oncologist may prescribe medications to take at home before chemotherapy, sometimes called *premeds*. These are usually given to prevent allergic reactions or other complications. You should also receive prescriptions and instructions for medications to take after treatment. Ask about how and when to use anti-nausea medications, pain relievers, or stool softeners, since both constipation and diarrhea are common during chemotherapy. Having these instructions clearly written out and stored in your cancer binder makes them easy to follow when you are at home. Some patients even create a chart with medication names, times, and checkboxes to mark each dose.

WORKBOOK CHECKPOINT: Turn to page 9/4, **My Pre-Meds and At-Home Medication Guide** in your workbook. Work with your oncology team to fill in this page with specific instructions for medications to take before and after chemotherapy. Having this written out clearly (including doses, timing, and purpose) prevents confusion when you're at home and not feeling well. Use your Planner to keep notes on symptoms and efficacy of the medications during your first few cycles to identify patterns, just like Laura did with her anti-nausea plan. This documentation helps your team make adjustments that improve how you feel.

It is also important to keep an updated list of every medication you take, including vitamins, supplements, and over-the-counter remedies. As you may recall, we began this list in Chapter 3, workbook page **My Current Medications and Allergies**. Bring it with you to appointments so your oncologist can review it. Certain supplements, especially in high doses, may interfere with chemotherapy, and your team will guide you on what is safe to continue.

One item that belongs on this list and is frequently left off is cannabis, in any form. Many patients do not mention it because it feels separate from their medical care or because they worry about being judged. It is not separate, and there is no judgment here. Cannabis is processed by the same system in your liver that handles many cancer drugs, which means it can affect how your medications work. Tell your oncologist before your first treatment begins. There is much more on this topic, including new research, in Chapter 15.

We also reviewed in Chapter 3 how to use your calendar or planner. Have one ready before your first infusion. Use it to record treatment dates, medications you take, and any side effects that you experience. Writing these down in real time allows your team to make adjustments more easily. For example, if nausea is consistently worse in the evenings, your oncologist may adjust the timing of your anti-nausea medications or add a new one. These changes are easier to make when symptoms are well documented with the date and time in your planner. Even small adjustments in medication can make a big difference in how you feel.

Patient Spotlight: Laura

Laura is my patient with Stage III endometrial cancer. Like many others, she came to her first consultation with a tote bag filled with pill bottles. She was taking several prescription medications, a handful of over-the-counter remedies, and a long list of supplements suggested by friends. At first, she felt uneasy when I asked her to go through them one by one, but once everything was written down, she admitted to feeling calmer. Having a complete list allowed us to sort out what was safe, what might interact with chemotherapy, and what truly helped.

Initially, Laura was reluctant to keep a planner. She insisted she would "just remember" when she felt nausea or became constipated. By her second infusion, however, she realized that recalling the details was harder than she had expected. She began writing down notes about when her symptoms occurred and what medications she took. At her next visit, the record helped us adjust her anti-nausea plan. Laura tells me that although writing everything down feels tedious at times, it gives her a sense of control and helps her feel like an active partner in her care.

What to Bring on the First Day of Chemotherapy

Your first chemotherapy infusion can feel overwhelming, but preparing a small *treatment day bag* ahead of time can make the experience more comfortable and less stressful. The goal is to bring items that help with both physical comfort and emotional support.

Wear loose-fitting, soft clothing and shoes that are easy to take on and off. If you have a port, choose a shirt that allows easy access to the chest area. Apply lidocaine cream to the port site before arriving, as it numbs the skin and lessens discomfort during access.

Bring a trusted companion if possible. Having someone there can provide emotional support, take notes, or simply keep you company during the long hours of treatment.

It's also wise to pack items that pass the time and help you relax. Light snacks, a water bottle, reading material, or an e-reader are popular. Many patients bring a favorite blanket or small pillow to make the infusion chair feel less clinical. Others use journals or planners to jot down thoughts, questions, or early side effects.

If you plan to use cryotherapy (ice packs or frozen gloves and socks) to protect your hands and feet from neuropathy, or cold capping to preserve hair, then be sure to bring the necessary supplies and a small cooler filled with ice or cooling bricks. A pair of headphones and a playlist loaded with music or podcasts can also be a welcome distraction. And don't forget a charger for your devices, so you are not left with dead batteries in the middle of the day.

WORKBOOK CHECKPOINT: Turn to page 9/5, **First Treatment Day Pack Checklist** in your workbook. Use this page to pack your day bag the night before your first infusion and check off each item as you pack it. This simple act reduces morning-of stress and ensures you don't forget anything important. After your first treatment, you'll develop your own rhythm and know exactly what you want to bring. Many patients keep a dedicated chemo bag packed with their favorite items, ready to grab and go for each appointment.

Remember, preparation is not about achieving perfection; it's about reducing stress and creating space for your body to heal. You've done the work, and you are ready!

Chapter 10

Treatment Day: What Really Happens and How to Feel Ready

Understanding Your Treatment Day

Treatment days often stretch into a full day, and the more you know about what to expect, the easier it is to walk in with confidence instead of fear. Understanding the step-by-step process can take away much of the mystery and help you feel more prepared and less anxious.

> **WORKBOOK CHECKPOINT:** Your workbook contains a **Treatment Day Flow Guide** on page 10/1. This page summarizes each step of your infusion appointment, from check-in to discharge. After reading this section, you can fill in the timing and details of your treatment day, which should help reduce anxiety. After your first treatment, add notes about what helped and what you would do differently next time.

Arrival and Check-in

Your day begins at the oncology department or infusion center, where you check in with the front desk staff. They will confirm your information, verify insurance, and may have you complete some paperwork. This is also a good time to ask about the schedule for the day and double-check that nothing has changed from what you were previously told.

Blood Work and Vital Signs

Before anything else, a nurse or medical assistant will check your vital signs: blood pressure, heart rate, temperature, and breathing rate. Your height will be measured at least once, and your weight will be checked regularly. These numbers matter. Chemotherapy doses are based on your height and weight, so if you've gained or lost more than ten pounds, tell your team so they can make sure the calculation is accurate. Weight changes also give clues about how you are eating, drinking, and whether you might be retaining fluid—all of which are important for your doctor to know.

Next comes blood work. A sample may be taken from a vein or from your mediport, if you have one. Sometimes, if only a complete blood count (CBC) is needed, a quick finger stick will do. These tests check your blood counts, kidney function, and liver function to make sure your body is ready for treatment. If the results show that your blood counts are too low, for example, platelets under one hundred thousand or neutrophils under one thousand, your treatment may need to be delayed or adjusted. In some cases, additional medications or transfusions are given first to get you safely back on track.

Patient Spotlight: Maria

Maria arrives for her third chemotherapy treatment feeling prepared and ready to get it over with. After her labs come back, however, her nurse tells her that her white blood cell count is too low and the infusion must be postponed. Maria feels frustrated since she took the day off work, arranged childcare, and mentally geared herself up to push through. At first, she is angry and disappointed, convinced that the delay will ruin her progress.

We take a few minutes to go over her labs together, and I explain that her body needs time to recover before the next dose. ***A short delay like this is very common and rarely changes the overall outcome of treatment.*** *Once Maria understands this, she admits that the stress of rearranging her schedule is real, but she also feels reassured that the delay is meant to protect her.*

Over time, she learns to expect the unexpected on treatment days. Sometimes it is blood counts, sometimes it is pharmacy delays, sometimes a machine breaks down. Instead of letting every detour drain her, Maria focuses on saving her emotional energy for the challenges that truly matter. She tells me later, "I realized I can't control the small stuff, but I can control how much power I give it."

Consultation with Healthcare Provider

Before proceeding to the treatment room, you may meet with your oncologist or an advanced practice provider such as a nurse practitioner or physician assistant. This visit is your opportunity to talk openly about how you are doing both physically and emotionally. It is also the best time to raise questions about your treatment plan, your side effects, or anything else on your mind.

Some patients feel pressure to put on a brave face and say everything is fine, even when it isn't. Please don't do this. Your team cannot help you if they don't know what you're struggling with. Bring your calendar or planner with you and use it to share details about side effects and how well your medications have worked. Even small notes like *Nausea worse at night on day two* or *Constipation lasted three days after chemo* can help your doctor fine-tune your treatment plan.

As doctors, we are trained to pick up on clues such as changes in your labs, weight, or vital signs, but we cannot know exactly what you are experiencing unless you tell us. When you share openly, it allows us to act quickly. Sometimes that means adjusting medications to better control nausea, prescribing an appetite stimulant, or giving treatment for fluid buildup if your body is holding on to more than it should.

Patient Spotlight: Lydia (Triple-Negative Breast Cancer)

When my patient Lydia came for her third infusion, she looked pale and tired. When I asked how she had been doing, she quickly said, "I'm fine." After reviewing her labs and vital signs, I noticed she was mildly dehydrated, and her weight had dropped. When I gently pressed further, Lydia admitted she had been so nauseated that she could barely eat. She thought she should push through and didn't want to bother us.

Once she shared the details, we adjusted her anti-nausea medications and added hydration before her infusion and again a few days later. By her next visit, she felt markedly better. Lydia later told me that speaking up felt uncomfortable at first, but once she did, she realized how much easier her treatment became.

> PLANNER REMINDER: This consultation step is why your **Cancer Journey Planner** matters so much. As Lydia discovered, documenting symptoms between appointments—*Nausea was worse on day two, couldn't keep down food on day three*—gives your team specific information to adjust your care. Vague descriptions lead to vague solutions. Detailed tracking leads to targeted help. Bring your planner to every consultation and review it together with your provider.

Pre-Infusion Checks

Before any medications are started, the nursing staff will go through a series of safety steps. Each time you are about to receive medication or undergo a procedure, you will be asked to state your full name and date of birth. This may feel repetitive, but it is one of the most important safeguards to ensure accuracy in your care.

Your nurse will then review your allergies, your home medication list, and any new symptoms or concerns since your last visit. They will also ask whether you experienced any side effects or adverse reactions with your previous chemotherapy. This information helps the team anticipate and prevent complications.

Next, you will receive the *pre-meds* that are given before chemotherapy, either by mouth or through your IV. These usually include a steroid such as dexamethasone, an antihistamine such as diphenhydramine (Benadryl), and an anti-nausea medication, such as aprepitant or ondansetron (Zofran). Hydration with IV fluids may also be given if needed.

If you are using a cold-capping system to help preserve hair, the cap is usually applied during this period so it has time to cool your scalp before chemotherapy begins.

Patient Spotlight: Emily

Emily, who was being treated for ovarian cancer, came to her infusion ready for treatment. About halfway through her pre-meds, she suddenly felt an odd sensation in her legs. She could not stop moving them and worried something serious was happening. The nurse explained that this was a reaction to the Benadryl she had received, a side effect called restless legs. Emily admitted she wished she had known this was a possibility, so she would not have panicked. After that visit, we talked through what she might feel with each pre-medication so she would be better prepared. Her team also switched her to a different antihistamine, so she did not have the same reaction again. Knowing what to expect and knowing that adjustments could be made helped Emily stay calm during future treatments and gave her the confidence to speak up quickly if something felt off.

> **PRO TIP:** If you experience unusual side effects with a pre-medication, let your team know. In many cases, alternatives can be used.

Chemotherapy Infusion

The main event of the day is the chemotherapy infusion itself. The length of time you spend in the chair depends on the drug regimen you are receiving.

Some infusions may be as short as thirty minutes, while others can take several hours. Your nurse will review the plan with you before starting, so you know what to expect.

During the infusion, you will usually be seated in a comfortable recliner in a treatment room. Depending on the setup at your center, you may be alongside other patients or in a private space. Nurses will check on you regularly to monitor how you are tolerating the medications. If you experience symptoms such as flushing, shortness of breath, itching, or nausea, let your nurse know right away. These may be signs of an infusion reaction, and the team is trained to respond quickly if they occur.

Some regimens require continuous medication over twenty-four to forty-eight hours. In that case, you may go home with a small infusion pump connected to your mediport. Your nurse will explain how the pump works and give instructions on what to do if you have questions or concerns while at home.

Most patients find that once the infusion is underway, the process is less intimidating than they imagined. This is a good time to use the comfort items you brought, such as snacks, water, a journal, headphones, or simply a blanket, to help you feel at ease.

WORKBOOK CHECKPOINT: Turn to page 10/2, **Recognizing and Reporting Symptoms During Infusion** in your workbook. This is a safety reference card. Review it and bring it to your infusion appointment to discuss with your infusion nurse. Emily's story shows why immediate reporting matters. Her nurses were prepared and responded quickly because she spoke up right away. Don't wait and don't minimize. Your team wants you to report symptoms immediately, even if you're not sure they are significant.

Monitoring and Support

The chemotherapy oncology nurses play a crucial role in your care, especially during your chemotherapy infusions. They will monitor your physical reactions closely and are available to support you if side effects such as nausea or discomfort occur. Make sure to communicate openly with them about how you are feeling at any point. If you experience any unusual symptoms, alert your nurse right away so you can be evaluated promptly.

Allergic reactions can occur even if you have received the drug before. Some drugs, like paclitaxel, are more likely to cause reactions early in the infusion. Others, such as carboplatin, may trigger a reaction later on. A reaction can begin with symptoms such as feeling your face get hot, itching (including on the palms of your hands), back discomfort, stomach pain, feeling the need to defecate, chest tightness, sudden nausea, or dizziness. In rare cases, reactions may escalate to shortness of breath, swelling, or a rapid heartbeat.

Your nurses are trained to pause the infusion, assess your symptoms, and give treatments such as antihistamines, steroids, epinephrine, or oxygen if needed. If a reaction happens, it can feel frightening, but your team is experienced and prepared to respond quickly to keep you safe. **Also, remember that severe reactions are uncommon.** In recent reviews of commonly used drugs such as taxanes, severe reactions occurred in only about 1 to 2 percent of patients despite premedication, although the exact risk varies by drug. While these events are uncommon to begin with, the vigilance of your care team adds an important extra layer of safety (Barroso et al. 2024).

Patient Spotlight: Emily (Ovarian Cancer)

During the first five minutes of Emily's second infusion of paclitaxel, she suddenly felt her face flush and her chest tighten. She panicked, convinced something terrible was happening. The nurse immediately stopped the infusion, called over a colleague, and started oxygen. Within moments, she received medication through her IV, and the nurses calmly explained that this was a reaction they see and manage often. Her symptoms eased within minutes, and she sat quietly while the nurses monitored her until she felt steady again. At her next treatment, Emily admitted she was still nervous, but she told me she felt safe knowing that her team recognized the problem quickly and knew exactly how to handle it.

Post-Infusion Care

Once your chemotherapy infusion is complete, you will not be sent home right away. Nurses will continue to monitor you for a short period to make sure you feel well enough to leave safely. Your vital signs are checked again, and you will be asked about any new symptoms before discharge.

If you have a mediport, the needle is carefully removed, the site cleaned, and covered with a small dressing. This process is called de-accessing, and once it is done, you can resume normal activities such as showering or light movement.

Before you go, your nurse will review instructions about what to expect over the next few days. This includes common side effects to watch for, which symptoms require a call to your doctor, and what steps to take if you feel unwell outside of office hours. You should also leave with your follow-up schedule clearly outlined, including your next infusion date, lab work, and any interim appointments with your oncologist.

It is normal to feel a mix of relief and fatigue after treatment. Some patients go home and rest immediately, while others feel well enough to resume light activity. Listen to your body and give yourself permission to recover in whatever way feels right for you.

> TRACK IT IN YOUR PLANNER: After each treatment, try to take five to ten minutes to reflect in your Cancer Journey Planner. Document things like:
>
> - How you felt during the infusion (physically and emotionally)
> - What comfort strategies worked (music, breathing, companion's presence)
> - What you'll do differently next time
> - Any questions that came up for your next appointment

Mindfulness Practices to Relieve Anxiety During Chemotherapy Sessions

For many patients, sitting through chemotherapy is not just a physical challenge but an emotional one. The setting can feel overwhelming, especially amidst the sound of infusion pumps, the sight of other patients receiving treatment, and the uncertainty of how your own body will respond. Anxiety is a natural reaction, but it can make the day feel longer and more difficult.

Mindfulness practices are simple techniques that help you stay present and calm. They do not erase the reality of chemotherapy, but they can give you a sense of control over how you experience it. Even a few minutes of focused breathing or guided imagery can lower stress, reduce muscle tension, and help you leave the infusion center feeling steadier than when you arrived.

Focused Breathing

One of the simplest yet most powerful mindfulness techniques is focused breathing. By paying deliberate attention to each inhale and exhale, you can slow down your body's stress response and create a sense of calm, even in the middle of an infusion.

To practice:

- Sit back in your chair and, if comfortable, close your eyes to minimize distractions.
- Inhale slowly through your nose for a count of four.
- Hold the breath gently for a moment.
- Exhale through your mouth for a count of four, letting your shoulders drop as you release tension.
- Repeat for several minutes, keeping your attention on the steady rhythm of your breath.

Patients often tell me this simple practice helps them manage racing thoughts and physical symptoms of anxiety, like a fast heartbeat or restlessness.

It can be done quietly without drawing attention and works well alongside other relaxation tools, such as listening to calming music or guided meditations through headphones.

Body Scan Meditation

Body scan meditation is another tool you can use to calm both mind and body. It involves paying close attention to physical sensations, from head to toe, and gently releasing areas of tension as you notice them. This practice can help you feel more grounded and less focused on worries about treatment.

To practice:

- Settle into a comfortable position in your infusion chair. Close your eyes if you wish.
- Take a few slow breaths to center yourself.
- Begin by focusing on the top of your head. Notice any sensations—warmth, tightness, or even nothing at all.
- Slowly move your attention downward, scanning each part of your body: face, shoulders, arms, chest, abdomen, legs, and finally your feet.
- As you reach each area, imagine tension melting away with each exhale.

Some patients describe this as a way of *checking in* with themselves. It helps them shift attention away from the busy infusion room and toward their own inner state, leaving them calmer and more in control.

Guided Imagery

Guided imagery is a technique that uses your imagination to bring about a sense of calm. By picturing a safe, peaceful place, you can shift your focus away from the infusion chair and into a setting that feels restorative.

To practice:

- If possible, use headphones to listen to a guided recording. Many apps and websites offer scripts that walk you through the process.

- If you prefer, guide yourself. Close your eyes and imagine a place where you feel completely at ease—a quiet beach, a forest trail, or even a favorite spot from your childhood.
- Engage all your senses. Notice the sights, sounds, smells, and textures. Is there sunlight on your skin? The sound of waves? The scent of pine?
- Allow yourself to linger in that space, letting your body relax as if you were truly there.

Patients often tell me that guided imagery helps them feel less like *a patient in a chair* and more like themselves again, connected to the parts of life that treatment cannot take away.

Mindful Listening

Mindful listening is a way to anchor yourself in the present moment by tuning into the surrounding sounds. Rather than letting noises in the infusion center feel distracting or irritating, you can use them as a focus point to calm your mind.

To practice:

- Sit quietly and notice the sounds around you—the gentle beeping of monitors, the hum of conversations, the footsteps in the hallway.
- Instead of reacting to these sounds, simply acknowledge them. Imagine each one passing by, like leaves floating down a stream.
- If you prefer, bring headphones and listen to calming music, nature sounds, or a favorite podcast. Give your attention fully to the sound, letting it carry you away from anxious thoughts.

Patients often say this practice makes the treatment room feel less clinical and more manageable. By shifting your relationship with sound, you transform the environment from something overwhelming into something you can coexist with peacefully.

Patient Spotlight: Emily (Ovarian Cancer)

After her reaction to paclitaxel, Emily admitted that she dreaded sitting down for her next infusion. The thought of it happening again made her anxious even before she walked into the center. We talked about simple mindfulness practices she could try during treatment. She chose mindful listening. With headphones on, she played a playlist of soft piano music and focused on each note. Later, she told me, "The music gave me something else to pay attention to instead of my fear of another reaction."

WORKBOOK CHECKPOINT: Turn to page 10/3: **Mindfulness Practices for Chemotherapy Sessions** in your workbook. This handout summarizes these skills and provides you with an easy cheat sheet you can bring with you to treatment appointments. Remember: you don't need to master every technique. Find what works for you and put the others aside.

Chapter 11

Between Treatments: Your Practical Guide to Recovery and Protection

Managing the Intervals Between Chemotherapy Sessions

The time between chemotherapy sessions is just as important as the treatment days themselves. How you recover at home can affect whether your next treatment happens on schedule. If your body has not bounced back enough, chemotherapy may need to be delayed. That is normal and sometimes necessary, but there are many ways you can support your recovery and lower the chances of setbacks. This chapter focuses on what to do and what not to do between cycles. We will review rest, hydration, medications, food choices, infection precautions, and some of the most common reasons treatments get delayed.

Returning Home After Chemotherapy: Managing Your Recovery

Rest and Recovery

Once you get home from chemotherapy, your main job is recovery. Fatigue is one of the most common side effects, and it often shows up in the first few days after treatment. Listen to your body and rest when you need to, even if that means napping more than usual. At the same time, avoid falling into a *couch potato* pattern. Gentle movement is good for your body and your mood. Aim for a balance: get up, walk around the house, stretch a little, then rest again. Small bursts of activity followed by breaks often work better than either constant rest or constant activity.

Patient Spotlight: Anna

Anna, an attorney, was determined not to let cancer slow her down. After her first infusion, she tried to keep her usual schedule, sitting at her desk for hours and pushing through her exhaustion. Within a day, she felt completely wiped out and frustrated with herself. At her next treatment, we made a new plan: instead of fighting her fatigue, she alternated light activity with rest. She found that short walks around her apartment, followed by a nap or quiet time, left her feeling stronger. Anna later admitted that pacing herself actually gave her back more energy than forcing herself to push through.

> TRACK IT IN YOUR PLANNER: Use your **Cancer Journey Planner** to document your energy patterns day by day. After a few cycles, you'll see your personal rhythm: *I'm always most tired on days two to three*, or *My energy returns by day seven.* This self-knowledge helps you plan activities, work schedules, and when to ask for help.

Staying Hydrated

Water is one of the simplest but most powerful tools for recovery. After chemotherapy, your body works hard to process the drugs and clear them from your system. Staying well-hydrated helps your body function better and may lessen symptoms such as fatigue, headache, and nausea.

Try to make water your main drink. For many people, **sixty-four ounces of fluid a day** is a reasonable starting goal, although you may need more if you are losing fluids or having trouble eating and drinking. Tea, coffee, and other beverages can still count toward your fluid intake, but plain water is usually the best choice. If water does not appeal to you, try adding a splash of juice, slices of lemon, lime, or cucumber, or choose herbal tea, diluted broth, or sugar-free flavored water.

> TRACK IT IN YOUR PLANNER: Set a daily fluid goal with your physician and record your intake as you go. Some patients like to fill water bottles in the morning and track how many they finish by the end of the day. A simple way to check your hydration is to look at your urine color. Pale yellow usually means you are on the right track.

Increase your fluid intake if you develop vomiting or diarrhea. Think of it as replacing what your body is losing. Please call your oncology team if you are unable to drink enough to meet this goal, if you feel weak and lightheaded, cannot keep liquids down, or have vomiting or diarrhea lasting more than twenty-four hours. Sometimes the solution is a better anti-nausea regimen, but sometimes you may need IV fluids to catch up. There is no shame in asking for that help. It can make a big difference in how you feel and keep you safely on track for your next cycle.

Managing Medications: Nausea and Bowel Movements

The medications you take at home after chemotherapy are just as important as the treatment itself. They are there to control side effects and help your body recover.

Nausea is one of the most common concerns, and the best approach is to be proactive. Two of the most prescribed anti-nausea medications are ondansetron and prochlorperazine, although I prefer prescribing ondansetron because, overall, I find it to be more effective. Do not wait until you are very nauseated to take your medication. Take it at the first hint of queasiness so it does not snowball into something harder to manage. On the other hand, there is usually no need to take anti-nausea drugs around the clock if you are feeling well. The key is to respond early.

Some patients need more than one medication to get full relief. In my practice, we often add medications such as prochlorperazine (Compazine), metoclopramide (Reglan), or olanzapine at bedtime, or even a short course of steroids like dexamethasone after treatment. These are usually introduced in later cycles if ondansetron alone does not provide complete control. If your nausea is severe despite taking ondansetron as prescribed, call your oncologist's office right away. Do not wait until your next appointment because adjustments can and should be made quickly.

Bowel changes are also common. Many patients become constipated right after treatment, often because of anti-nausea medications like ondansetron. A few days later, diarrhea may hit when the constipation breaks, often triggered by taking multiple laxatives to reverse it. To prevent this rollercoaster, I often recommend taking a gentle laxative such as polyethylene glycol (MiraLAX), senna, or magnesium hydroxide (milk of magnesia) in the evening after chemotherapy. For many patients, this simple step prevents the worst constipation and avoids the rebound diarrhea that follows.

> TRACK IT IN YOUR PLANNER: Log your daily nausea and bowel movements in your planner using workbook page 11/1: My Recovery and Symptom Management Plan as a guideline.

Patient Spotlight: Laura

After her first chemotherapy treatment, Laura became constipated and, feeling uncomfortable, tried several laxatives in succession. The next day, she developed diarrhea that left her feeling weak and uneasy. She called the clinic, and we brought her in for IV hydration to help her recover. For her next cycle, we made a proactive plan: she took a single, gentle laxative the evening after chemotherapy. This prevented both constipation and rebound diarrhea, and she told me it made her feel much more in control.

UPDATE YOUR MEDICATION LIST: Add all new prescriptions to your **Current Medications and Allergies** page 3/2 from Chapter 3. Include anti-nausea medications (Zofran, Compazine), laxatives (MiraLAX, senna), and any new additions from your team. I recommend that you try to keep this list current and bring it to each appointment.

Dietary Considerations After Chemotherapy

Food can be both a comfort and a challenge after chemotherapy. What you eat matters for recovery, but so does how you eat. Many patients find that appetite changes, nausea, or altered taste make eating feel like work. Small, frequent meals are often easier than three larger ones, and lighter foods can be gentler on your stomach in the first days after treatment. Broths, yogurt, oatmeal, scrambled eggs, mashed potatoes, and smoothies are good starting points if you feel unsettled.

Maintaining your weight is an important goal during treatment, though what that means can vary depending on your situation. If you are receiving chemotherapy with the goal of preventing cancer from coming back (adjuvant treatment), the focus is on staying nourished without gaining unnecessary extra weight. Comfort foods, such as carbohydrates, are understandable, but be mindful that calories still count, and excess weight gained during treatment will need to be addressed later.

For patients with more advanced cancer, the priority shifts to preventing weight loss and making sure every bite provides value. Protein becomes especially important to help with healing, immune function, and strength. Good sources include chicken, fish, eggs, beans, lentils, tofu, and dairy products. If solid foods are difficult, smoothies or nutritional shakes can be an easier way to get protein. A practical minimum goal is about one gram of protein per kilogram of body weight per day, and many patients may benefit from more if they can tolerate it. For example, a 75 kg person would aim for at least seventy-five grams of protein daily. If this feels overwhelming, a consultation with a nutritionist or oncology dietitian can help translate that goal into realistic meals and snacks that fit your appetite and preferences.

Nutrition in oncology is a complex topic, and this is only a brief overview. Overall, try not to be discouraged if your appetite changes from day to day. Try eating small, frequent meals to help maintain your blood sugar levels, which in turn will help keep your energy and strength up. And most importantly, reach out to your oncology team if you need guidance.

Nutrition Between Treatments

Between treatments, eating becomes less about perfection and more about staying strong enough to keep going. Treatment can change appetite, digestion, and immune function. My goal in this section is to help you make safer choices, reduce avoidable complications, and keep your energy as steady as possible. If you are struggling to eat or drink for more than a day or two, tell your oncology team. There is a point where food strategies are not enough, and you need medical support.

Should You Avoid Sugar When You Have Cancer?

The concern about sugar and cancer stems from the fact that cancer cells, like all cells in your body, use glucose, which is a type of sugar, for energy. Some people worry that eating sugar will directly *feed* the cancer and make it grow faster. While that idea is scary, the relationship between sugar and cancer is much more complex (Makarem et al. 2018).

We all know that, in general, eating a diet high in sugar is not good for us. The more complicated question is how much sugar and what type of sugar matter the most while you are actively in treatment. High sugar intake can contribute to weight gain and insulin resistance. Those are not just long-term issues. They can affect how stable you feel during treatment and may shape the broader metabolic environment, which promotes cancer to grow (Makarem et al. 2018).

The concern about sugar is not simply about *feeding* cancer. Instead, the stronger evidence points to the metabolic effects of high-sugar dietary patterns, including weight gain, insulin resistance, and activation of growth-signaling pathways. All cells, including cancer cells, need sugar (glucose) for energy, but restricting sugar in your diet does not selectively starve cancer cells without also depriving healthy cells of necessary fuel.

A better explanation for why sugar matters is the pattern of sugar spikes in the bloodstream. Diets high in sugar can lead to increased inflammation and insulin resistance. High blood sugar levels increase insulin production, which signals the liver to increase production of insulin-like growth factor 1, or IGF-1. That is normal biology. The catch is that IGF-1 has been shown in laboratory models to stimulate cancer cell growth and survival, particularly in cancers of the breast, colon, and lung (Davison et al. 2011), (Kasprzak 2021), (Yeo et al. 2017). Avoiding large sugar spikes helps keep IGF-1 levels steadier. That is why limiting a high-sugar diet may be a reasonable supportive strategy during cancer treatment, even though it is not a cure by itself (Davison et al. 2011).

Practically, I often recommend a low-glycemic approach. Foods are chosen because they are nutritious and less likely to cause large spikes in blood sugar and insulin. The key is to maintain a balanced diet with complex carbohydrates and fiber, so your body still produces energy, but in a more controlled and even tempo. This is a supportive nutrition strategy, not a stand-alone cancer treatment (Treasure et al. 2021).

Practical Tips (Sugar Without the Fear)

- **Limit sugary beverages and snacks:** Cut back on sodas, candies, and baked goods, which offer little nutritional value and are frequently high in glucose or other simple sugars.

- **Choose whole foods:** Opt for whole fruits instead of fruit juices or sugary snacks. Whole fruits provide fiber, vitamins, and minerals. Fiber slows the absorption of sugar, which is why it is healthier to eat an apple than to drink a glass of apple juice.
- **Watch for hidden sugars:** Be aware of added sugars in processed foods like cereals, sauces, and packaged snacks. Read labels carefully.

In summary, there is no need to eliminate sugar from your diet completely. Focus on a balanced, nutrient-rich diet with complex carbohydrates and fiber. If you want individualized guidance, ask your team to connect you with a registered dietitian familiar with oncology care.

Food Safety Between Treatments (When Your Immune System Is Not at Full Strength)

Chemotherapy can weaken your immune system and can also cause side effects that affect how well you can eat and digest food. During treatment, food safety matters more than usual. The following sections describe some foods that I recommend my patients try to avoid during chemotherapy because they may carry a higher risk of infection and are often not worth the gamble. If your team has told you that you are neutropenic (more susceptible to bacterial infections), or if you have had recent infections, take these precautions even more seriously. In many cases, the goal is not an overly restrictive *neutropenic diet*, but careful attention to safe food handling and avoiding higher-risk foods.

Raw and Undercooked Foods

One of the most important precautions during chemotherapy is to avoid raw and undercooked foods. These foods can harbor harmful bacteria and parasites, which pose a greater risk when your immune system is compromised. Raw meat, pork, poultry, and seafood should be cooked to recommended internal temperatures. Raw eggs and foods containing raw eggs, such as homemade mayonnaise, Caesar dressing, and some desserts like tiramisu, should be avoided. Sushi and sashimi are also risky due to contamination from raw fish. Unpasteurized dairy products can contain harmful bacteria, so choose pasteurized milk, cheese, and other dairy items.

Unwashed Fruits and Vegetables

Fruits and vegetables are a vital part of a healthy diet, but during chemotherapy, you need to handle them with extra care. Unwashed raw fruits and vegetables can carry bacteria, dirt, and pesticide residue. Wash them thoroughly under running water before eating, cutting, or peeling. Firm produce can also be scrubbed with a clean vegetable brush. Some people choose to use a brief, diluted white vinegar soak for produce that will be eaten unpeeled. Small studies suggest this may help reduce some surface bacteria and pesticide residue, but plain running water remains the standard recommendation (Alreshoodi et al. 2024).

Salads and raw sprouts, such as alfalfa, clover, and radish sprouts, are particularly prone to contamination and are best avoided unless thoroughly washed. For those with more significant immune suppression, cooking the vegetables can provide an additional layer of safety and is often easier on the digestive system.

Foods with a High Risk of Contamination (And Why I Care About This One)

During cancer treatment, your immune system is often compromised, making you more vulnerable to foodborne infections. Deli meats and processed meats are particularly problematic. They carry an immediate contamination risk and a longer-term cancer concern.

First is the infection risk. Deli meats can be contaminated with *Listeria monocytogenes*, a harmful bacterium that poses a serious threat to anyone with a weakened immune system. Research shows that Listeria can cause more severe illness in people with cancer, especially those receiving immune-system-suppressing therapy, than it does in the general population (Snellings et al. 2025). For that reason, if you are going to eat deli meats during treatment, the safest approach is to avoid them or heat them until steaming hot before eating. Better yet, during the active treatment phase, it may be wisest to skip them entirely.

The second concern extends beyond your immediate treatment. In 2015, the World Health Organization classified processed meats as Group 1 carcinogens. That includes bacon, hot dogs, sausages, and deli meats. This does **not** mean they are as dangerous as tobacco or asbestos. It means the evidence linking processed meat to cancer is considered convincing (Bouvard 2015).

Why does this matter? Processing methods such as curing and smoking can create cancer-causing compounds, including N-nitroso compounds. The clearest link is with colorectal cancer. Eating just fifty grams of processed meat a day—about one hot dog or a few slices of deli meat—has been associated with about an 18 percent increase in colorectal cancer risk (Bouvard 2025). An association with stomach cancer has also been observed, although that evidence is less conclusive (Bouvard 2015).

The bottom line is that processed meats carry both immediate infection risks during treatment and long-term cancer risks afterward. I recommend avoiding them altogether. Choose freshly cooked chicken, turkey, fish, or plant-based proteins instead. Your body needs real nutrition right now, not chemicals and preservatives, and certainly not Listeria.

Eating for Tolerance (When Your Gut Is Not Cooperating)

High-Fiber and Gas-Producing Foods

Fiber is generally healthy, but during chemotherapy, certain high-fiber foods can exacerbate diarrhea or gas. If you are sensitive, use them in moderation. Limiting beans, lentils, whole grains, and high-fiber fruits and vegetables can help manage these symptoms. Gas-producing foods such as beans, broccoli, and cabbage are often better tolerated when cooked rather than eaten raw. Carbonated beverages, such as sodas or even seltzers, can cause bloating and discomfort and may be best avoided if you notice they trigger symptoms.

Foods and Beverages That Can Cause Mouth and Throat Irritation

Chemotherapy and other anti-cancer treatments can cause mouth sores and throat irritation. Certain foods and beverages will make these symptoms worse. Spicy foods, acidic foods and drinks such as citrus fruits, tomatoes, and vinegar-based foods, and extremely hot foods and beverages should be avoided. Allow foods to cool to a moderate temperature before consuming to prevent further irritation.

If you do experience mouth sores or difficulty swallowing, opt for soft, easy-to-digest foods like yogurt, smoothies, mashed potatoes, and soups.

Infection Risk in Cancer Patients Receiving Chemotherapy

An important thing to understand about chemotherapy is that it unfortunately does not only target cancer cells. It also decreases activity in the bone marrow, which is where white blood cells are created. When white blood cells decline, especially neutrophils, it becomes much harder for the body to fight infection. The most urgent warning sign is a fever. A temperature of 100.4°F (38.0°C) or higher is never ignored in a patient on chemotherapy or certain other targeted treatments that cause low white blood cells. Fever can be the first and sometimes only sign of infection, and it always deserves a call to your oncology office right away. While some treatments themselves can trigger fever unrelated to infection, it is still essential to report these episodes in real time so your medical team can determine next steps.

Neutropenic Fever

Neutropenic fever is a potentially life-threatening complication of chemotherapy. It refers to fever in the setting of a very low white blood cell count (an absolute neutrophil count [ANC] less than 1.0). Because the immune system cannot mount a strong response, infections can spread quickly and may become serious before typical signs like pus or redness appear. For this reason, most patients with neutropenic fever are admitted to the hospital for intravenous antibiotics until the source is clarified and blood counts recover.

Fortunately, medications called growth factors have decreased the frequency of severe complications. Drugs such as filgrastim (Neupogen) or the longer-acting pegfilgrastim (Neulasta) stimulate the bone marrow to produce more neutrophils and are often built into regimens known to carry a high risk of neutropenia. The downside is that these shots can cause bone pain. Antihistamines such as loratadine (Claritin), NSAIDs like ibuprofen or naproxen, acetaminophen, or even short-term narcotics may be used to ease this discomfort.

Where and How Infections Arise

Infections in chemotherapy patients do not always come from an obvious outside source. Chemotherapy can damage the lining of the mouth, stomach, and intestines, creating openings where normal bacteria can enter the bloodstream. Tumors themselves can also obstruct normal pathways such as the bile ducts, intestines, or the urinary tract, making infections more likely. In addition, the underlying cancer can impair the immune system even before treatment begins.

Patient Spotlight: Emily

Emily, one of my patients with ovarian cancer, taught me how quickly things can change. About ten days after treatment, she called the after-hours on-call physician with a fever of 100.6°F. She had no cough, no sore throat, and no urinary symptoms. However, it is common for patients not to have any other symptoms that would typically point to an infection, at least not initially. Because she was on chemotherapy, she was directed straight to the hospital, where they drew blood cultures and started intravenous antibiotics right away. Fortunately, her fever resolved and her counts recovered within a few days. She was sent home with oral antibiotics, and her next treatment was only delayed a few days. Emily later told me that the scariest part was how suddenly it happened and how if she had not known to call, she might have just taken Tylenol and gone to bed. She was very glad that she had listened to the instructions and recovered so uneventfully.

Strategies to Avoid Hospitalization

While hospitalization is sometimes unavoidable, there are steps you can take to reduce the risk of infection and stay on track with treatment.

Vaccinations play a critical role. Before starting chemotherapy, ask your oncologist if you are up to date on the influenza vaccine, pneumococcal vaccine, and shingles vaccine (Shingrix). These can prevent serious secondary infections and help avoid treatment delays.

Hygiene is simple but powerful. Wash your hands often, especially before meals and after using the bathroom or coming home from public places. Hand sanitizer is an effective backup when soap and water are not available.

Dietary precautions also matter. Avoid raw or undercooked meats, seafood, and eggs, as well as unpasteurized dairy. Wash fruits and vegetables carefully—I often recommend a diluted white vinegar rinse and gentle scrub to remove bacteria and pesticides. Use deli meats within four to five days of purchase. Sushi and other raw fish are best avoided during chemotherapy due to the risk of bacterial contamination.

Environmental controls can decrease exposure to viruses. Clean frequently touched surfaces such as doorknobs and counters, and try to avoid close contact with sick individuals or large indoor crowds during peak viral seasons.

Viral infections deserve special mention. Chemotherapy patients remain susceptible to viruses such as influenza, RSV, and COVID, which can be harder to recover from and can also trigger secondary bacterial infections, such as catching the flu and then developing bacterial pneumonia. For this reason, I often recommend wearing a mask in crowded public spaces. An extra layer of protection may make a difference in reducing setbacks.

Prophylactic medications are rarely used but may be prescribed in high-risk situations. These include preventive antibiotics or antifungal drugs, usually reserved for patients with extremely weakened immune systems.

And most importantly, **report symptoms promptly**. Fever, chills, sore throat, burning with urination, or anything unusual should trigger a call to your oncology team. I generally advise calling the oncology office first rather than a primary care walk-in clinic, since your oncology team knows both the risks of your specific regimen and how aggressively infections need to be treated.

Conclusion

Protecting yourself from infection is one of the most important things you can do between chemotherapy treatments. Even small precautions can make a big difference in lowering your risk, such as washing your hands often, being mindful of what food you are eating, or wearing a mask in crowded places. Remember, a fever of 100.4°F (38.0°C) or higher is always a reason to call your oncology office immediately. Staying alert and reporting symptoms quickly allows your team to act before problems become serious. These steps not only safeguard your health but also help ensure that your treatment stays on schedule.

WORKBOOK CHECKPOINT: For a quick reference guide on what to do (and what to avoid) between treatments, see the companion workbook pages 11/1 and 11/2.

Chapter 12

Managing Common Side Effects: The Practical Solutions That Actually Help

Side effects are one of the hardest parts of cancer treatment. They can make you miserable in the moment, but they also matter for the bigger picture. If nausea, fatigue, or pain keep you from eating, sleeping, or showing up for treatment, it can throw off the entire schedule. And with cancer care, staying on track often means better results.

The good news is that most side effects can be managed. There are medications, tricks, and supportive therapies for almost everything you will face. What you should never do is suffer in silence. Telling your doctor or nurse how you really feel is not complaining; it is giving them the information they need to help you.

In the pages that follow, I'll walk you through the side effects I see most often: hair loss, bone pain, constipation, dehydration, diarrhea, heartburn, leg swelling, nausea, neuropathy, and watery eyes. I'll explain why they happen, what you can do about them, and when it's time to pick up the phone and call the office. My goal is not to overwhelm you with lists, but to give you enough practical knowledge so that when something comes up, you're not blindsided. You'll know what's happening, and you'll know you have options.

Alopecia (Hair Loss) During Chemotherapy

Hair loss is one of the side effects patients dread most. Not every chemotherapy causes it, but when it does, it usually starts about two to three weeks after the first dose. Drugs like doxorubicin, paclitaxel, and docetaxel (when given every three weeks) almost always cause complete hair loss. Other drugs such as carboplatin, cyclophosphamide, fluorouracil, and gemcitabine may only cause thinning. Knowing what to expect helps you prepare mentally. Some patients will choose to shave their scalps to avoid the emotional trauma and physical inconvenience of their hair falling out. This is a completely personal choice.

As discussed in Chapter 9, cooling caps can sometimes help. These are worn during chemotherapy and work by chilling the scalp. The cooling causes constriction of the blood vessels, so less chemotherapy drug reaches the hair follicles to cause damage. They are not effective for all regimens, and not everyone finds them tolerable.

Your scalp deserves gentle care. Use mild shampoos and light moisturizers. Some women develop folliculitis, an inflammation of the hair follicles, during shedding. This can be treated with topical clindamycin or, if severe, an oral antibiotic.

Think ahead about head coverings. Wigs, hats, and scarves can soften the blow. A lot of my patients like to purchase a soft cotton head wrap to wear at night or when lounging. They make it more comfortable and less drafty when sleeping or when you are not wearing your wig. Your oncologist's office should have resources, and a national directory of free wigs, hats, and scarves for cancer patients can be found at cancercarenews.com/more-cancer-freebies/hats-wigs-scarves. Further resources can be found in the workbook.

Eyelashes and eyebrows may fall out with prolonged chemotherapy, although not everyone experiences this. They will grow back, and over-the-counter remedies like castor oil or other cosmetic lash growth serums applied with a small brush can help speed the process. There are also bimatoprost drops (Latisse), which require a prescription but are usually not covered by insurance.

Hormonal anti-estrogen therapy does not usually cause complete hair loss, but thinning is common. Anti-estrogen drugs can cause hair to shed gradually over time. Gentle care still applies here, and some patients use topical Rogaine or oral supplements like Nutrafol, but make sure to discuss with your own oncologist because there are differing opinions regarding their use.

The bottom line is that losing your hair is awful… Okay, *it sucks*! But there are ways to prepare, soften the impact, and support regrowth. More importantly, talking about how you feel matters because this is not just cosmetic. Your hair is part of your identity, and your care team should help you through it.

Bone Pain

Bone pain during cancer treatment is not one-size-fits-all. It usually comes from treatments like paclitaxel or anti-estrogen therapy, sometimes from supportive medicines like G-CSF (Growth Factor Support: a protein that stimulates the bone marrow to produce more white blood cells), and less often from the cancer itself spreading to the bone. Each situation requires its own approach.

Treatment Side Effects (Paclitaxel, Hormonal Therapy)

Taxane chemotherapy, particularly paclitaxel, can trigger an acute pain syndrome with muscle and joint aches. These pains often show up a few days after a dose and usually fade within a week. Scientists believe the cause is nerve sensitization or irritation in the spinal cord. Nothing shows on imaging, but patients feel it clearly.

Hormonal therapies, especially aromatase inhibitors, can also cause deep, achy bone or joint pain. The sudden loss of estrogen affects bone remodeling and puts a strain on joints and tendons. Patients often describe this as stiffness and soreness that feels different from regular arthritis.

Growth Factor Support (G-CSF)

G-CSF is used to help your bone marrow recover after chemotherapy by stimulating white blood cell production. It lowers infection risk and keeps treatment cycles on schedule. The downside is that this rapid bone marrow expansion stretches the marrow cavity and causes dull, nagging aches. These pains can be intense for a few days but are usually manageable with supportive medication.

Bone Metastasis

The least likely cause, but the most serious in a patient receiving adjuvant (preventative) treatment, is if the cancer has spread to the bone. When this happens, the bone weakens, normal repair is disrupted, and fractures may result. A fracture that happens because of cancer is called a pathological fracture. Pain from bone metastases requires more complex interventions, including bone-strengthening drugs, the possibility of radiation therapy for the pain or to stabilize the bone, and sometimes braces or surgery for stability.

Management Strategies

Treatment depends on the cause. For chemotherapy or hormonal therapy aches, over-the-counter medicines such as ibuprofen (Advil, Motrin), naproxen (Aleve), or acetaminophen (Tylenol) are often effective.

A typical regimen that I will suggest for G-CSF pain includes:

- Naprosyn 500 mg every twelve hours by prescription, or Aleve two tablets every twelve hours over the counter, starting the morning after the injection and continuing for five days. This medication might not be recommended for someone with an allergy to NSAIDs, on a blood thinner, or with a history of peptic ulcer disease, or even with poor kidney function. Please check with your doctors to ensure that you can take NSAIDs (non-steroidal anti-inflammatory medications).

- Omeprazole (Prilosec) 20 mg at bedtime to protect the stomach while taking these medicines.
- Loratadine (Claritin) 10 mg daily for five days after the injection (Kirshner et al. 2018).
- Tylenol Arthritis (or generic) two tablets every twelve hours if needed.
- Oxycodone (a narcotic requiring a prescription) only if the pain remains severe.

For bone metastases, we often combine bone-strengthening drugs such as bisphosphonates or denosumab with radiation and physical therapy. These treatments can relieve pain, lower fracture risk, and improve mobility.

When to Worry

If your bone pain is sharp, worsening over time, or accompanied by swelling, redness, or pain that does not ease with medication, contact your doctor. These could be signs of a fracture or infection and need immediate attention.

Constipation

Constipation is one of the most common and frustrating side effects patients face during cancer treatment. It can happen for many reasons: chemotherapy itself, pain medications like opioids, anti-nausea medicines, or simply reduced activity and fluid intake. The bowels slow down, stools become harder, and the effort to pass them can be painful and downright exhausting.

Why It Happens

Chemotherapy and anti-nausea medications can disrupt the normal movement of the intestines. Pain medications, especially opioids, directly slow down the gut by binding to opioid receptors in the digestive tract. Reduced activity and lower food, fiber, and fluid intake during treatment make the problem worse. For some patients, constipation can become severe enough to require hospital treatment if not managed early.

Management Strategies

Hydration

Fluids are the foundation. Aim for at least sixty-four ounces of water daily unless your doctor has told you otherwise. Warm liquids like coffee or tea can also stimulate bowel activity.

Exercise

Gentle activity, such as walking or light stretching, helps stimulate the intestines. Even short walks a few times a day can make a noticeable difference.

Diet

Include fiber-rich foods like fruits, vegetables, and whole grains. Fiber helps bulk up the stool, but it only works if you are drinking enough fluids. Without fluids, added fiber can make constipation worse.

Medications

When lifestyle measures are not enough, medications can help:

- **Bulk-forming laxatives** (such as psyllium) absorb water and add bulk to stool, but they require consistent fluid intake, i.e., drinking a lot of water.
- **Stimulant laxatives** (such as senna or bisacodyl) speed up intestinal activity. They act quickly, though sometimes at the cost of cramping. They also have a rebound effect: if used every day for long periods, the intestines can become lazy, making bowel movements harder once the medicine is stopped. For this reason, stimulant laxatives are best used for short-term relief, not as a daily solution.
- **Osmotic laxatives** (such as polyethylene glycol/MiraLAX or lactulose) draw water into the intestines to soften stool. They are effective for persistent constipation but can cause bloating.

- **Magnesium laxatives** (such as milk of magnesia) pull water into the colon and usually work within hours. This is one of my favorite remedies because it is fairly gentle and does not usually cause cramping like some other medications can. It also comes in liquid and tablet form.
- **Stool softeners** (such as docusate sodium) help mix water into stool, making it easier to pass. These are gentle and particularly helpful if straining is a concern. However, a review published in 2021 found that docusate was no better than a placebo for stool softening (McRorie et al. 2021). Nevertheless, they are still very commonly used and are very gentle, so you can decide for yourself.
- **Lubricant laxatives** (such as mineral oil) coat the intestines and stool, helping retain moisture. These can be given as an enema, but enemas are generally discouraged in immunocompromised patients due to infection risk.
- **Prescription medications**, such as lubiprostone (Amitiza) and linaclotide (Linzess), may be needed for patients with opioid-induced (from pain medications containing narcotics), refractory constipation, or irritable bowel syndrome with constipation.

Practical Advice

Try to remember to track your bowel movements in your planner, including what you took to help and the results. This record helps your care team adjust medications and avoid trial-and-error guessing. Do not ignore constipation for more than a few days, especially if you feel bloated, nauseated, or unable to eat.

PRO TIP: If you received ondansetron (Zofran) as part of your chemotherapy, consider taking a gentle laxative the evening you return home. Ondansetron is very effective for nausea, but it also slows down the gut, and constipation can set in quickly. Taking a laxative that night often allows you to have a bowel movement the following day and keeps things moving before the problem snowballs.

If you are using stimulant laxatives, be aware of the rebound effect. Your intestines may move well while you are taking them, but once you stop, things can slow down again, sometimes even more than before. This is normal, but it means stimulant laxatives should be used with care and not as your only tool. Pair them with hydration, diet, and gentler options like stool softeners or osmotic laxatives so you are not relying on stimulants alone.

The Bottom Line

Constipation is uncomfortable, but it is best managed with early attention. Fluids, gentle movement, diet, and the right medicines can keep it from derailing your treatment. Most importantly, stay ahead of your symptoms and let your oncology team know if you are having trouble so they can help you find relief.

Dehydration

Dehydration is one of the most dangerous yet overlooked problems during cancer treatment. Your body is already under stress from chemotherapy, radiation, or the cancer itself, and losing too much fluid can quickly tip you into a medical emergency.

Why It Happens

There are several reasons why dehydration is so common in cancer patients. Treatments often reduce appetite and make drinking fluids less appealing. Nausea and vomiting directly deplete fluids, and diarrhea can strip your body of both water and electrolytes in a matter of hours. Fever, which is more likely when your immune system is suppressed, increases fluid loss through sweat while also lowering the desire to drink. When dehydration sets in, your blood pressure can drop, your kidneys can become stressed, and the body's ability to process chemotherapy weakens.

Management Strategies

The single most effective step is increasing fluid intake. Water is best, but diluted juices, herbal teas, or broth may be easier to tolerate if plain water feels unappealing. Many patients find it easier to sip a few ounces frequently rather than forcing down a large glass all at once. Oral rehydration solutions such as Pedialyte, DripDrop, Liquid IV, or Hydralyte are excellent choices because they replace electrolytes as well as fluids. Just as important is managing the underlying causes: taking anti-nausea medication so you can keep liquids down, and controlling diarrhea promptly to avoid large losses. In some cases, despite your best efforts, intravenous fluids may be needed. This is common and should not be seen as a failure but rather as a safe and effective way to restore hydration quickly.

Practical Advice

One of the simplest habits that makes a big difference is tracking your fluid intake the way you would track your medications. Marking off bottles or recording ounces in your planner shows you right away if you are falling behind. If you find you are unable to drink enough, do not wait until you are dizzy, confused, or barely urinating to alert your care team. At that point, dehydration is much harder to reverse. Instead, report these issues early so small interventions can prevent a larger problem.

The Bottom Line

Dehydration is a common complication from chemotherapy, but a relatively easy one to tackle. Staying well hydrated protects your kidneys, keeps your treatments on schedule, and helps you feel stronger day to day.

Diarrhea

Diarrhea during cancer treatment can be tricky to manage. Some patients swing between constipation and diarrhea depending on the medicines they are taking. In my practice, I define diarrhea as three or more loose bowel movements in a twenty-four-hour period. I do not usually recommend starting medication after a single episode unless it is persistent or there is a clear pattern.

Why It Happens

Chemotherapy, radiation to the abdomen or pelvis, and certain targeted therapies can all irritate the lining of the gut. These treatments make it harder for your intestines to absorb water, which leads to loose stools. Anti-cancer drugs can also disrupt the balance of bacteria in your gut, further worsening the problem.

Management Strategies

The first step is controlling symptoms, and the most commonly used medication is loperamide (Imodium), which is available over the counter. You can take it following the directions on the package; the usual dosage is two tablets after a loose bowel movement, and then one tablet after each subsequent loose bowel movement. I am often more conservative in the beginning and recommend taking one tablet after you have had two or three loose bowel movements and then continue with one tablet after each subsequent bout of diarrhea.

If diarrhea continues, prescription medications such as diphenoxylate-atropine (Lomotil) can be used. For severe or stubborn diarrhea, your oncologist may even prescribe octreotide, which can be given as a subcutaneous injection, by IV, or oral liquid.

Maintaining hydration is just as important as stopping the diarrhea itself. Every episode means fluid and electrolyte loss. Water is essential, but oral rehydration solutions, as discussed above, are often better because they replace both fluids and salts and can be purchased on Amazon or from most pharmacies.

Dietary changes help too. Eat small, frequent meals instead of three large ones. Bland foods such as bananas, rice, applesauce, and toast are easier to digest and less likely to make diarrhea worse. Avoid high-fiber foods, raw fruits and vegetables, greasy or fatty meals, spicy dishes, and dairy if they seem to trigger symptoms.

Practical Advice

Keep notes in your planner of your bowel movements, what you ate, and what medicines you tried. This log helps your team figure out the best approach for you going forward. If you develop irritation from frequent stools, clean the area gently and use barrier ointments or wipes such as Preparation H wipes, Preparation H cream, or Doctor Butler's ointment. Another option is to take a warm bath with some Epsom salt or purchase a sitz bath to soak your bum in. If irritation persists, contact your physician's office for a topical steroid and/or a topical anesthetic.

Most importantly, **know when to call your oncologist**. Do not wait this out on your own if any of the following occur:

- Diarrhea with three or more loose stools a day lasting more than three days despite over-the-counter treatment
- Signs of dehydration, such as dizziness, headache, or dark urine
- Fever, severe abdominal pain, or vomiting
- Feeling too weak to keep up with fluids on your own

The Bottom Line

Diarrhea is disruptive and very bothersome, but it can be managed. Stay hydrated, use medicines wisely, and call your oncology team promptly if red-flag symptoms appear.

Heartburn

Heartburn, also called acid reflux, is a burning discomfort in the chest or throat that many patients experience during cancer treatment. It is common, uncomfortable, and if ignored, it can interfere with eating and sleeping, which are obviously two things you need to do well during treatment.

Why It Happens

Cancer treatments themselves often set the stage for reflux. Chemotherapy, targeted drugs, and certain pain medicines can irritate the lining of the esophagus. Steroids, which are commonly given with chemotherapy, increase acid production. Treatments may also slow digestion, allowing stomach contents to linger and back up more easily. For patients with fluid in the abdomen (ascites), the extra pressure can make reflux worse.

Some people are predisposed to heartburn even before cancer therapy. The lower esophageal sphincter (LES), the muscle that normally acts as a one-way valve between the stomach and esophagus, can malfunction. This may happen because of defective nerve control, impaired smooth muscle function, or a hiatal hernia, where part of the stomach protrudes through the diaphragm. Risk factors that increase reflux include obesity, pregnancy, certain diets (fatty or spicy foods, chocolate, caffeine), alcohol and tobacco use, eating large meals, or lying down too soon after eating. Many common medications can also relax the LES and worsen symptoms.

How to Manage It

Lifestyle changes can make a big difference. Try eating smaller meals more often instead of three large ones. Avoid trigger foods such as chocolate, caffeine, spicy dishes, tomatoes, citrus, alcohol, or greasy meals if you notice they make symptoms worse. Do not lie down for at least three hours after eating, and try elevating the head of your bed by six to eight inches so gravity can help keep stomach contents down while you sleep. One way to do this is with extra pillows or a foam wedge. Another option is to raise the entire head of the bed with a few bricks strategically placed under the bed frame. Of course, make sure to mention your plan ahead of time if you share your bed with someone else.

If these new habits and physical changes do not do the trick, then medication will help most people. The following are in order of strength and efficacy:

- *Antacids* like Tums or Maalox neutralize stomach acid quickly but only work for a short time. (As a bonus, Tums also provides a source of calcium.)
- *H2 blockers* such as famotidine (Pepcid) reduce acid production and last longer. Pepcid Complete combines an antacid like Tums for fast relief with an H2 blocker for longer control.
- *Proton Pump Inhibitors (PPIs)* such as omeprazole (Prilosec) and esomeprazole (Nexium) are stronger, but they take longer to work and can interfere with the absorption of other medicines or electrolytes if used long term.

Practical Advice

Keep a symptom diary. Write down what you ate and when the heartburn happened. That way, you can spot your personal triggers instead of guessing. If you have ascites and your heartburn suddenly worsens, ask your doctor if draining the fluid (a procedure called paracentesis) is appropriate.

Also, do not add new medicines on your own without talking to your team. Some cancer drugs interact with common acid reducers, and it is important that your oncologist knows what you are taking.

Call your oncology team right away if you notice:

- Trouble swallowing or feeling like food is stuck in your chest
- Vomiting blood or material that looks like coffee grounds
- Black or tarry stools
- Heartburn that does not improve despite using medicines as directed

The Bottom Line

Heartburn may feel minor compared to other side effects, but if it is not controlled, it can wear you down. Small changes in diet, the right medications, and open communication with your care team will usually keep it under control.

Leg Swelling

Leg swelling, or edema, is a common issue that cancer patients may encounter for various reasons. It's essential to understand the causes and management strategies to help alleviate this uncomfortable condition.

Common Causes of Leg Swelling in Cancer Patients

Lymphedema

Lymphedema happens when lymph nodes are damaged or removed during cancer treatment, or when radiation scars the lymphatic channels. With fewer drainage pathways, lymph fluid has nowhere to go and collects in the tissues, usually in the arms or legs. Patients describe the swelling as heavy and uncomfortable, and it may not go away with simple measures like elevation.

Lymphedema can appear weeks, months, or even years after treatment. Once it develops, it is often chronic and requires ongoing management. The best way to control it is with manual lymphatic drainage performed by a trained lymphedema therapist, followed by consistent use of compression garments to prevent fluid from reaccumulating. Left untreated, lymphedema can worsen over time, increase the risk of infection (cellulitis), and interfere with daily activities.

Medications

Several cancer therapies and supportive medicines can cause leg swelling by promoting fluid retention. Chemotherapy drugs such as docetaxel and gemcitabine are known culprits. With docetaxel in particular, swelling can be significant, and pretreatment with oral steroids is often used to reduce this side effect. Some hormonal therapies can also contribute to fluid buildup.

It is not just cancer drugs—commonly used blood pressure medications, especially amlodipine (Norvasc), can cause swelling as well. Steroids given during chemotherapy can temporarily worsen edema, too, though the effect is usually reversible once the steroid is tapered.

When medication is the cause, swelling often improves once the drug is stopped or changed. In cases where the medication must be continued, your oncology team may use supportive strategies such as diuretics, compression stockings, or steroid premedication to help control the problem.

Decreased Activity and Poor Diet

Being less active can cause fluids to accumulate in your legs because muscle action helps pump fluid back up to your heart. This is particularly notable when you're not eating enough protein in your diet. Protein in your diet is measured in your blood by albumin, and gives your doctor an indication of how well you're eating and/or absorbing your food. Low albumin in the blood allows fluids to leak out into the skin (edema). If your albumin level is low in your bloodwork, your doctor may make dietary recommendations, add medication to increase appetite, and perhaps send you to see a nutritionist.

Blood Clots

Cancer patients are at a higher risk of developing blood clots, which can block blood flow and cause swelling. A clot in the leg or pelvis, called a deep vein thrombosis (DVT), is a serious condition and usually requires treatment with blood thinners. The most dangerous complication is when part of the clot breaks off and travels to the lungs, creating a pulmonary embolism (PE). A PE can be life-threatening, which is why it is so important to recognize and treat blood clots in the leg quickly.

One of the telltale signs of a DVT is when only one leg suddenly becomes more swollen than the other. The gold standard tests for diagnosis are a lower extremity Doppler ultrasound, which looks at blood flow in the veins, or a CT scan with intravenous contrast if a clot is suspected higher up in the pelvis.

Venous Insufficiency

Sometimes genetics, smoking, or simply aging can weaken the veins in your legs. When this happens, blood has a harder time returning to the heart and instead pools in the legs. The result is swelling, heaviness, and tenderness over the affected veins. This condition is usually chronic and less likely to come directly from cancer treatment, but it can show up during your care and make leg swelling worse.

There are often skin changes that go along with venous insufficiency. The veins may become enlarged and twisted, creating visible varicose veins. Smaller red or blue networks of veins, often called spider veins, may appear on the skin's surface. Over time, the skin around the ankles and lower legs can darken to a reddish-brown color. In later stages, the skin may also thicken, harden, and feel leathery, or become dry, flaky, and itchy.

Raising your legs, when possible, may bring temporary relief, but most patients benefit more from wearing compression stockings, which improve circulation and limit fluid buildup. If swelling and tenderness continue to worsen, a consultation with a vascular surgeon may be helpful to discuss other options.

Congestive Heart Failure (CHF)

Congestive heart failure is usually a chronic condition that develops when the heart cannot pump blood effectively due to damage to the heart muscle. When the heart's pumping ability weakens, blood backs up in the veins and fluid leaks into the tissues of the legs and feet, causing peripheral edema (such as swelling in the legs). Patients often notice weight gain as fluid builds up throughout the body.

Certain chemotherapy drugs can increase the risk of heart failure. Doxorubicin is the most well-known. It can cause congestive heart failure in about 7 percent of patients, but this risk is dose-dependent and usually occurs once a lifetime cumulative dose of 550 mg/m^2 is reached. Therefore, a lifetime dose is always monitored when a patient is on this medication. Trastuzumab can also cause heart failure, but in most cases, the changes are reversible once the drug is stopped. Because of these risks, patients receiving either of these drugs have intermittent echocardiograms (ECHO) to monitor heart function during treatment.

An echocardiogram is an ultrasound of the heart that measures its pumping strength, called the ejection fraction (EF). A normal EF is between 50 and 70 percent. Lower numbers mean the heart is not contracting as well as it should.

One clinical clue that swelling may be related to heart failure is that it often involves both legs, and it often improves overnight when the legs are elevated.

Cellulitis

Cellulitis is an infection of the skin and the tissues underneath. It causes swelling, redness, warmth, and pain in the affected leg. In cancer patients, the risk is higher because chemotherapy weakens the immune system, and lymphedema makes it easier for bacteria to take hold. The swelling from cellulitis often appears suddenly and is frequently accompanied by fever or chills.

This is a medical emergency. Cellulitis requires prompt antibiotics, sometimes given through an IV if the infection is severe. Left untreated, it can spread quickly and become life-threatening.

The Bottom Line

Leg swelling is common during cancer treatment, but it is not always harmless. Sometimes it comes from fluid retention, lymphedema, or weak veins, and other times it can signal something serious, such as a blood clot, infection, or heart failure. Paying attention to when the swelling started, whether it affects one or both legs, how it changes with rest or elevation, and whether there are other symptoms like redness, pain, or shortness of breath can help your team figure out the cause. Always let your oncology team know about new or worsening swelling so it can be evaluated and treated quickly.

Nausea

Nausea is one of the most feared side effects of chemotherapy. It can show up right away, linger for days, or even start before treatment if your body has learned to expect it (called anticipatory nausea). Poorly controlled nausea doesn't just make you miserable; it can stop you from eating, drinking, or even showing up for the next infusion. Fortunately, we have a wide range of medicines and supportive strategies to keep it under control. Here is a section so you can understand them.

Why It Happens

Nausea and vomiting during cancer treatment come from a complicated loop of signals between the gut and the brain. Chemotherapy irritates the stomach and intestines, releasing serotonin, which is a neurotransmitter that activates the vagus nerve. At the same time, drugs stimulate the brain's chemoreceptor trigger zone. Multiple neurotransmitters are involved, including serotonin, dopamine, substance P, histamine, and acetylcholine. This is why there are different anti-nausea medicines that target different chemical pathways in the body.

First, you need to understand that there are several distinct patterns of nausea, which are sometimes treated differently. *Acute nausea* appears within the first twenty-four hours of treatment and is usually driven by serotonin. *Delayed nausea* develops two to seven days later and is linked to substance

P. *Anticipatory nausea* can start before chemotherapy and is triggered by the sights, smells, or even just the memories of treatment. *Breakthrough nausea* occurs despite taking the medicine prescribed to prevent it, and *refractory nausea* continues despite multiple different treatments being used together.

How to Manage Nausea Associated with Treatment

Medications

5-HT3 Receptor Antagonists

Ondansetron (Zofran), granisetron (Kytril), and palonosetron (Aloxi) block serotonin receptors in the gut and the brain. This stops serotonin, which is released by chemotherapy, from activating the nausea and vomiting reflex. They work best for acute nausea that occurs within the first twenty-four hours of treatment. Side effects include headache and constipation. Because constipation is so common with ondansetron, I usually tell patients to take a gentle laxative the evening they get home from chemo so they do not get backed up the next day (see Constipation section).

NK-1 Receptor Antagonists

Aprepitant (Emend), fosaprepitant, and rolapitant block a chemical called substance P, which plays a major role in delayed nausea that can occur two to seven days after chemotherapy. By preventing substance P from binding to NK-1 receptors in the brain, these drugs reduce the likelihood of nausea that lingers long after treatment. They are generally well-tolerated but can interact with other medications, so it is important that your oncology team knows all the drugs and supplements you are taking.

Corticosteroids

Dexamethasone works on several levels to reduce inflammation and dampen the signals that cause nausea. It is often combined with other antiemetics to make them more effective. Dexamethasone is helpful for both acute and delayed nausea, but it can cause agitation, trouble sleeping, and higher blood sugar.

Olanzapine

Olanzapine is an antipsychotic medication that affects multiple brain pathways, including dopamine and serotonin. By blocking these signals in the brain's vomiting center, it works against acute, delayed, and breakthrough nausea. In my practice, it often reduces the need for steroids and ondansetron. The most common side effect is drowsiness, which is why I usually start with the lowest dose (2.5 mg) at bedtime.

Dopamine Antagonists

Prochlorperazine (Compazine), metoclopramide (Reglan), and promethazine block dopamine in the brain's vomiting center, which helps stop nausea that breaks through despite other medicines. Metoclopramide also improves stomach emptying, which can reduce the feeling of fullness or bloating. Side effects may include drowsiness, restlessness, or muscle stiffness, especially if these medicines are used often.

Benzodiazepines

Lorazepam (Ativan) does not directly block nausea signals. Instead, it reduces the anxiety and conditioned responses that cause anticipatory nausea—when your body reacts before chemo even starts. It also has a calming effect that can make nausea easier to tolerate. Side effects include sedation, balance problems, and forgetfulness, so it is usually prescribed in small doses.

Cannabinoids

Dronabinol and nabilone are synthetic versions of compounds found in cannabis and are FDA-approved prescriptions to treat nausea and loss of appetite. They act on cannabinoid receptors in the brain to reduce nausea and sometimes improve appetite. These drugs are not considered first-line, but they can help with refractory nausea that does not respond to other medicines. Side effects include dizziness, confusion, or feeling *high*. It is important to distinguish these medications because they are not the same as cannabis products purchased at a dispensary, which vary widely in strength and how they are compounded, and are also not regulated as medications. If you are using or considering commercial cannabis for symptom management, please discuss it with your oncologist before your next treatment. There is important information about cannabis and breast cancer treatment covered in Chapter 15 that is worth reading before making that decision.

Integrative and Complementary Approaches to Nausea

Lifestyle and Diet

Simple changes can make a real difference. Eat smaller, more frequent meals instead of three large ones. Spicy, greasy, or heavy foods often make nausea worse, while bland foods like bananas, rice, applesauce, or toast are usually gentler. Staying hydrated is just as important. Sip clear fluids throughout the day and aim for at least sixty-four ounces unless your doctor advises otherwise.

Integrative and Complementary Approaches

Several non-drug strategies can support your care. Ginger (about one gram daily) has been shown to reduce acute nausea. Acupressure or acupuncture at the P6 point on the inner wrist helps some patients. Aromatherapy with peppermint oil, chewing gum, or sucking on lemon can ease nausea triggered by smells. Relaxation techniques, guided imagery, and music therapy can also help, especially with anticipatory nausea.

Practical Advice

The key is to take nausea seriously right away. Do not wait until you are miserable—start your anti-nausea medicine at the first sign of trouble. These drugs are not meant to be taken *just in case*, if you have no symptoms, unless your team specifically tells you to for a high-risk regimen.

If one drug isn't enough, your team may recommend alternating medicines, such as ondansetron every eight hours and prochlorperazine every six hours. This approach is only used if nausea isn't controlled with a single medicine, and it can be very effective.

If ondansetron is part of your regimen, remember it almost always causes constipation. Protect yourself by taking a gentle laxative the night you get home from chemo.

For patients with anticipatory nausea, I often recommend a small dose of lorazepam before treatment. It helps calm the conditioned response triggered by simply walking into the infusion room.

And one of the most important steps—document your nausea. Write down when it starts, what you took, and how well it worked. Bring that record to your next visit. It gives your oncology team and me the information we need to fine-tune your regimen instead of guessing.

The Bottom Line

Nausea is one of the toughest parts of chemotherapy, but it is also one of the most manageable. With the right medicines, simple adjustments in diet and hydration, and supportive techniques, most patients achieve good control. Stay ahead of your symptoms, write them down, and let your team know what is and isn't working so your plan can be adjusted.

Peripheral Neuropathy

Peripheral neuropathy refers to damage to the nerves outside of the brain and spinal cord. It is one of the more frustrating side effects of cancer treatment because it affects daily life in ways that are hard to ignore. Initial symptoms are usually numbness or a tingling sensation in the hands or feet, which can progress to a burning pain, sensitivity to touch, and, when severe, patients can develop weakness and loss of balance. Clearly, our best approach is to prevent these symptoms from developing altogether.

Why It Happens

Chemotherapy is the most common cause. Drugs such as cisplatin, carboplatin, paclitaxel, docetaxel, vinorelbine, bortezomib, and thalidomide are well known for damaging peripheral nerves. Radiation therapy can also injure nerves in the field being treated. In some cases, tumors themselves press on nearby nerves, or surgery may inadvertently damage them. Rarely, neuropathy develops as part of a paraneoplastic syndrome, when the immune system attacks the nervous system in response to cancer.

Some patients already have risk factors before treatment begins. Diabetes is one of the leading causes of peripheral neuropathy and can worsen symptoms once chemotherapy is added. Poor circulation from vascular disease, often seen in people with a history of smoking, also increases the risk. Vitamin deficiencies, including Vitamin D, B12, folic acid, and B6, can also damage nerves. Please note that many of the following recommendations are based on literature and research from patients with diabetes. Further defining the cause, treatment, and prevention of chemotherapy-induced peripheral neuropathy is an unmet need in oncology and requires more research.

How to Manage Peripheral Neuropathy

Medications

Anticonvulsants

Drugs like gabapentin (Neurontin) and pregabalin (Lyrica) are often first-line for neuropathy pain. They work by calming overactive nerves and stabilizing electrical signaling, which reduces pain and tingling. They do not help the neuropathy heal, but they work by stopping the signals that cause you to feel pain. These medications need to be adjusted gradually and monitored to find the right dose. Side effects include drowsiness, dizziness, and sometimes swelling in the legs.

Antidepressants

Certain antidepressants also help with nerve pain because of the way they alter neurotransmitters in the brain and spinal cord. Duloxetine (Cymbalta) and venlafaxine (Effexor XR) are commonly used serotonin-norepinephrine reuptake inhibitors (SNRIs). These medications can be used during the day and are less likely to cause sleepiness. Older tricyclic antidepressants like amitriptyline and nortriptyline can also be effective, though they sometimes cause dry mouth, constipation, or drowsiness.

Topical Treatments

Lidocaine patches can numb a painful area without affecting the whole body. Capsaicin cream, derived from chili peppers, works by depleting a chemical called substance P from nerve endings, which reduces pain signaling over time. Some patients also benefit from topical CBD (Cannabidiol), which may calm irritated nerves locally and reduce inflammation. Some preparations include a combination of agents such as menthol, topical anti-inflammatory drugs like arnica, as well as CBD.

Pain Relievers

For mild neuropathy, over-the-counter pain relievers such as acetaminophen or ibuprofen may help. For more severe pain, tramadol or oxycodone can be used, but opioids are generally reserved for short-term control because of side effects.

Supplements

Supplements are not a cure for neuropathy, but they can give your nerves the support they need to prevent, heal, and function better. I usually start my assessment by correcting any deficiencies. Vitamins B12, B6, and folic acid are essential for nerve health, and if you are low, symptoms can worsen. Some studies have shown that adding uridine nucleotides to the folic acid and Vitamin B12 may be effective in reducing nerve pain from peripheral neuropathy (Negrão et al. 2014). The levels of these vitamins can be measured in routine blood work and should be monitored, especially if you are on a supplement. High levels of folic acid have also been shown to increase some forms of neuropathy (Muhamad et al. 2023).

Some patients run into a different problem: their B12 level looks low, or their folate is off, even though they are taking in enough. In those cases, I sometimes test for MTHFR mutations with a simple blood test, which is available through most commercial labs. MTHFR (methylenetetrahydrofolate reductase) mutations are genetic variations that interfere with how your body processes folate and related pathways. If present, patients usually have better results on *methylated* forms of folate and B12, which bypass the genetic block and are easier for the body to use.

Vitamin D has been shown to play a role in diabetic neuropathy. Deficiency in Vitamin D is felt to contribute to both the development as well as the progression and worsening of peripheral neuropathy (Putz et al. 2022). Vitamin D levels can be measured in the blood as Vitamin D25-OH with a target range of 20-40 ng/mL, although there is some thought that higher levels (40-60 or even 70-80 ng/mL) may be beneficial for other metabolic functions (Grant et al. 2025). The precise level of Vitamin D is still under debate and should be discussed with your physician.

Alpha-lipoic acid is another option. This antioxidant has been studied in diabetic neuropathy, and I have seen it help patients on chemotherapy as well. The most common dose is 600 milligrams daily, usually on an empty stomach to improve absorption (Vallianou, Evangelopoulos, and Koutalas 2009).

Acetyl-L-carnitine, an amino acid, has shown benefit in studies of chemotherapy-induced neuropathy. I generally use doses in the range of 1,500 to 3,000 milligrams a day.

Omega-3 fatty acids from fish oil or flaxseed can also be helpful. A daily dose of one to two thousand milligrams of combined EPA and DHA supports the cell membranes that wrap around nerve fibers and reduces inflammation (Ko et al. 2010).

Magnesium is another mineral worth serious consideration. Certain chemotherapy drugs, such as carboplatin and cisplatin, as well as proton pump inhibitors for acid reflux, like Prilosec, cause the body to not absorb magnesium. Therefore, it is extra important to supplement if you are taking any of these medications. Magnesium helps calm overactive nerve signals and protects against the excess calcium that can build up inside nerve cells. Not all forms are created equal. I prefer **magnesium glycinate, malate,** or **threonate,** which are gentler on the stomach and better absorbed. Most adults benefit from 300 to 420 milligrams of elemental magnesium per day, though I recommend starting at the lower end and adjusting as tolerated.

PRO TIP: Always keep an updated list of your supplements and bring it to your oncology visits. A lot of patients forget to mention these, but it is important for your team to know exactly what you are taking so they can check for interactions, make sure you are using the right forms, and help you get the full benefit without unintended side effects.

Lifestyle and Supportive Care

Managing neuropathy is not just about prescriptions and supplements. Supportive measures can make the difference between struggling with symptoms and staying active and safe.

For patients with diabetes, keeping blood sugar levels well controlled (less than 110 mg/dL) is one of the most powerful ways to protect nerve health. Unstable or high glucose levels accelerate nerve damage and make chemotherapy-induced neuropathy worse. For smokers, quitting is critical. Smoking not only harms overall health, but it also reduces blood flow to the nerves, which starves them of the oxygen and nutrients they need to repair themselves. Some of my patients with the worst neuropathy have been those who did not quit smoking.

Specialists can also play an important role. A neurologist can perform detailed testing, monitor whether neuropathy is progressing, and recommend tailored treatments. Physical therapists focus on building strength, improving balance, and lowering the risk of falls. They can also help you re-learn safe walking patterns if sensation in your feet is reduced (I have seen this make a very big difference for some of my patients). Occupational therapists help with the day-to-day challenges that come with neuropathy—things like buttoning clothes, gripping utensils, writing, or using the computer. They can also teach techniques to improve fine motor skills and recommend adaptive tools when needed.

Simple adjustments at home can go a long way in preventing injuries. Non-slip mats in the bathroom and kitchen, sturdy handrails on stairs, and wearing shoes with good support all reduce the chance of falls. Good lighting is important too, especially if you have decreased sensation in your feet and need visual cues to stay steady. Patients who are experiencing weakness in the hands may benefit from kitchen tools and pens designed with larger, easier-to-grip handles.

Neuropathy may not always be preventable, although we should try. Nevertheless, these measures are aimed at making it more manageable. They also give you back some control, which is often what patients feel they are missing when symptoms creep in.

Eye Changes During Treatment

Eye problems are common during cancer therapy and can range from watery eyes to temporary vision changes. Most of these issues are not dangerous, but they can be uncomfortable and sometimes interfere with daily life. Recognizing the different causes is important because the right management depends on what is driving the symptoms.

Watery or Irritated Eyes

Chemotherapy can make the eyes water excessively, often because the eyes are actually dry and irritated. Some drugs inflame the surface of the eye or eyelids, which triggers more tear production. Others can block the tear ducts, the small channels that normally drain tears into the nose, so fluid builds up and runs down the face. The composition of tears may also change, making them less effective at lubricating the eyes. The body senses this and produces even more tears.

Not all tearing is chemotherapy-related. Allergies can also cause itchy, watery eyes, while infections tend to cause thicker discharge, redness, and sometimes pain or fever. It is important to recognize the difference because infections require immediate treatment. Certain newer treatments, such as Elahere (mirvetuximab), are also known to cause more serious eye irritation. Patients on these drugs should be followed closely by an ophthalmologist.

Blurry Vision

Blurry vision can develop for several reasons during treatment. Dry eyes may scatter light unevenly, leading to temporary blur. Corticosteroids like dexamethasone (Decadron), which are often used with chemotherapy, can cause fluid retention in the eye itself and lead to swelling that changes vision. These effects are usually temporary and resolve once the medication is stopped. I counsel patients not to rush out and change their eyeglass prescription if their vision shifts during chemotherapy, because in many cases the changes are reversible.

How to Manage It

For dryness and irritation, preservative-free artificial tears are usually the first step. Brands like Systane, Refresh, Blink, or generics are all good options. Warm compresses can help open tear ducts and reduce irritation. Sunglasses or protective glasses shield the eyes from wind and bright sunlight. Good hygiene and avoiding rubbing the eyes also help reduce further irritation or the risk of infection.

When to Seek Help

If watery eyes or blurred vision do not improve with simple measures, or if you develop redness, pain, thicker discharge, or vision changes that are severe or sudden, contact your oncology team. An ophthalmologist may prescribe medicated drops or perform procedures to open blocked ducts. For patients on drugs like Elahere, ophthalmology follow-up should be routine.

The Bottom Line

Eye changes during treatment are common and usually manageable. Most are temporary, whether related to chemotherapy, steroids, or dryness, but they should not be ignored. Supportive care with artificial tears, warm compresses, and eye protection can help with comfort. And if symptoms worsen, your care team can involve an ophthalmologist to make sure nothing more serious is happening.

WORKBOOK CHECKPOINT: As you add over-the-counter medications, symptom-relief drugs that you take as needed (PRN), or supplements to manage side effects, update your medication and supplement list from workbook Chapter 3/2. Also, as a reminder, track your daily symptoms and medication doses in your planner. Your medication list tracks what you are taking overall. Both tools matter and will help your oncology team to keep you safe and your symptoms well-managed.

Chapter 13

"How Many More Treatments, Doctor?": Understanding Your Timeline

In oncology, treatments are classified based on their timing and purpose in relation to the primary cancer treatment. This was discussed in Chapter 7, but here is a recapped overview of the differences between adjuvant and neoadjuvant treatments. I will also discuss the role of palliative treatments in the setting of metastatic cancer.

Adjuvant Treatment

Adjuvant chemotherapy is typically recommended after the main surgical intervention. The primary goal of surgery is to remove the visible tumor; however, microscopic cancer cells may linger, undetectable by scans or during surgery. Adjuvant therapy aims to eradicate these residual cells, thereby reducing the risk of cancer recurrence. The number of treatments and type of chemotherapy used in the adjuvant setting is decided based upon results of clinical trials, which determined the best dosing and number of cycles (treatments) for each cancer type. Thus, there is a predefined number of treatments.

Neoadjuvant Treatment

Conversely, neoadjuvant chemotherapy is administered **before** the surgical removal of the tumor. The primary aim here is to reduce the size of the tumor, making it more manageable for surgical removal and, in some cases, allowing for less extensive surgery. Again, in the breast cancer analogy, shrinking the main tumor in the breast might enable a lumpectomy instead of a more extensive surgery with a mastectomy. Neoadjuvant chemotherapy can also provide valuable insights into how the cancer responds to treatment. For instance, neoadjuvant therapy allows us to evaluate a tumor's response in real time. Usually, there are a predetermined number of treatments planned prior to surgery, but if a tumor does not show sufficient shrinkage in response to specific drugs, then therapy may be changed or additional treatments added prior to surgery to allow for more effective destruction of the cancer cells. In most cancer types, a patient will receive neoadjuvant chemotherapy followed by surgery, then receive further adjuvant therapy, and possibly maintenance therapy after that. More on maintenance therapies to come.

Treatment of Metastatic/Stage IV Cancer

The approach to treatment is different when the cancer has spread beyond the confines of where it began, i.e., to different organs or outside of the original regional lymph nodes. Therapy is considered palliative in this circumstance as it is not possible to cure the cancer in most cases (although there are some very limited circumstances where it is possible to put a patient into complete remission). Thus, the question, *How many more treatments, Doctor?* is much more difficult to answer in this situation. The truthful answer is that a patient with metastatic cancer will usually need to be on and off treatment for the rest of their lives, and there is no set number of treatments. The goals of chemotherapy for metastatic cancer are primarily aimed at three purposes:

- **Control the Cancer**: The primary goal is to shrink tumors, slow their growth, and prevent further spread. While curing metastatic cancer is often not possible, controlling the disease can extend a patient's life and improve quality of life.
- **Alleviate Symptoms**: By reducing the size and number of tumors, chemotherapy can help relieve symptoms caused by the cancer, such as pain, fatigue, and organ dysfunction.
- **Improve Quality of Life**: Effective chemotherapy can help patients feel better and maintain their daily activities and independence.

Additionally, palliative anti-cancer approaches may include a combination of modalities, including radiation therapy, surgery to relieve symptoms, medications to manage symptoms, as well as integrative approaches, such as acupuncture, massage, and relaxation exercises, which can help mitigate symptoms and improve well-being.

Patient Spotlight: Lisa

Lisa is a fifty-five-year-old woman with metastatic breast cancer who was experiencing severe pain due to bone metastases. Her palliative care team includes a pain specialist who prescribes a combination of pain medications and a palliative radiation oncologist who provides targeted radiation therapy to reduce the tumor size in her bones. Additionally, her medical oncologist gave her denosumab (Xgeva) injections to strengthen her bones and low-dose weekly paclitaxel chemotherapy. This combination helps manage her pain and control the pace of her disease, allowing Lisa to continue enjoying activities with her family.

Maintenance Therapy

After completing your primary cancer treatment, whether that was adjuvant chemotherapy, neoadjuvant therapy followed by surgery, or treatment for metastatic disease, you might hear your oncologist mention *maintenance therapy*. This term often confuses patients because it sounds like you will never truly *finish* your treatment. So, let me explain what maintenance therapy means in different situations, and why it has become such an important part of modern cancer care.

What Is Maintenance Therapy?

Maintenance therapy refers to ongoing treatment given after your initial therapy has achieved its goal. The purpose is to help prevent cancer from returning or, in the case of metastatic disease, to keep it under control for as long as possible.

Think of it like staying on blood pressure medication after your numbers improve. Although we are not treating active disease anymore, it is necessary to take the maintenance therapy to prevent it from coming back.

Unlike the intensive chemotherapy cycles you may have experienced, maintenance therapy is typically less toxic and more manageable. These treatments are often given as oral medications you take at home, or by injection/ intravenous infusions at periodic visits with your oncologist.

Why Doctors Recommend Maintenance Therapy

The concept behind maintenance therapy is straightforward. Cancer cells may be persistent and undetectable with our current methods of surveillance. Thus, even when scans show no evidence of disease and you feel well, microscopic cancer cells may still be present in your body. Maintenance therapy works to eliminate these remaining cells or keep them from growing and spreading.

The decision to recommend maintenance therapy is based on extensive research showing that certain medications can significantly reduce the risk of cancer recurrence and, in metastatic settings, extend the time before cancer progresses. Your oncologist will consider your specific type of cancer, the genetic characteristics of your tumor, your response to initial treatment, and your overall health when deciding whether maintenance therapy is appropriate for you. It is important to mention that the role of ctDNA monitoring may change the playing field of who should be recommended to receive maintenance therapy. More on this later in the chapter.

Common Examples of Maintenance Therapy

PARP Inhibitors as Maintenance

For patients with BRCA mutations or certain types of ovarian cancer, PARP inhibitors like olaparib or niraparib may be recommended as maintenance therapy after they have responded well to chemotherapy (O'Malley et al. 2023), (Tew et al. 2020). The key word here is *after*. You have completed your chemotherapy cycles, your scans show a good response, and now we use the PARP inhibitor to help maintain that response. These medications exploit the cancer's faulty DNA repair mechanisms to prevent regrowth.

It is important to understand that PARP inhibitors can also be used as an active treatment in other situations, such as for patients with BRCA mutations and metastatic breast cancer (Daly et al. 2024). But in the maintenance setting, we are using them specifically to keep cancer from returning after a good response to initial therapy.

Immunotherapy Maintenance

In certain cancers, particularly some types of lung cancer and triple-negative breast cancer, immunotherapy agents like pembrolizumab (Keytruda) may be continued as maintenance therapy after you have responded to initial treatment. The goal is to help your immune system continue recognizing and attacking any remaining cancer cells.

Targeted Therapy Continuation

Patients with HER2-positive breast cancer typically continue trastuzumab (Herceptin) and sometimes with pertuzumab (Perjeta) for a full year as part of their treatment plan. This medication blocks the HER2 protein that fuels certain breast cancers. We are not treating active disease at this point. We are preventing it from returning.

Bevacizumab Maintenance

In ovarian cancer, bevacizumab (Avastin) may be continued as maintenance therapy after responding well to initial chemotherapy. One mechanism by which this medication works is by preventing tumors from forming new blood vessels that they need to grow.

Hormone Therapy in the Adjuvant Setting

This one gets a bit complicated because hormone therapy serves different purposes depending on your situation. In early-stage breast cancer, if you have completed curative treatment and your cancer is estrogen receptor-positive, you may take tamoxifen or an aromatase inhibitor for five to ten years. This is classic maintenance therapy. We are preventing hormone-sensitive cancer cells from receiving the signals they need to grow.

The key difference here is timing and intent. This hormone therapy comes after you have completed your primary treatment (such as chemotherapy), *or* it is the primary treatment with the intention to cure the cancer. This is different from hormone therapy used to actively treat metastatic disease, where the breast cancer cells are still present, because in this scenario, there is no defined period of time to remain on the treatment.

How Long Does Maintenance Therapy Last?

This is one of the most common questions patients ask, and the answer varies significantly depending on your situation. Some maintenance therapies have defined endpoints based on extensive research. For example, hormone therapy for breast cancer is typically prescribed for five to ten years because clinical trials have shown this duration provides the maximum benefit in preventing recurrence. Others, particularly in metastatic disease, may continue indefinitely as long as they are working and you are tolerating them well.

Your oncologist will monitor your response to maintenance therapy through regular examinations, blood work, and imaging studies. If the therapy stops working or if you develop intolerable side effects, your treatment plan will be adjusted accordingly.

The bottom line is this: the duration is not arbitrary. It is based on what research has shown works best to keep you cancer-free.

Understanding the Side Effects

Maintenance therapies are generally much more tolerable than the intensive treatments you may have received initially. However, they are not without side effects. Because these medications are often taken for extended periods, managing long-term side effects becomes particularly important.

Common side effects vary by medication type but may include fatigue, joint pain, hot flashes, digestive issues, or an increased risk of infections. The key is open communication with your healthcare team about any symptoms you experience. Often, side effects can be managed effectively with supportive care measures or dose adjustments.

You are not expected to suffer in silence. Please advocate for yourself and discuss the side effects with your oncology team.

When Maintenance Therapy Is Recommended

Not every patient needs maintenance therapy, but when your oncologist recommends it, there is usually compelling evidence that it will significantly improve your chances of staying cancer-free. Your oncologist will evaluate your cancer type and stage, genetic markers, response to initial treatment, and overall health to determine if maintenance therapy is appropriate.

For many patients, particularly those with hormone receptor-positive breast cancer or BRCA-mutated ovarian cancer, maintenance therapy is considered a critical part of achieving a long-term cure. The research showing benefit is often so strong that most oncologists consider it standard of care, not an optional treatment.

Questions to Ask Your Oncologist

When maintenance therapy is recommended for you, consider asking these questions:

- What specific benefit does this maintenance therapy provide for my type and stage of cancer?
- What does the research show about outcomes with and without this therapy?
- How long would I need to take this medication?
- What are the most common side effects, and how can they be managed?
- How will we monitor whether the therapy is working?
- What are the risks if I choose not to take this medication?

Living with Maintenance Therapy

Many patients find that maintenance therapy allows them to return to a more normal life while continuing to actively prevent cancer recurrence. Unlike chemotherapy cycles that may have disrupted your routine for months, maintenance therapy can often be integrated into your daily life with minimal disruption.

The psychological aspect of maintenance therapy varies among patients. Some find great comfort in continuing active treatment, knowing they are doing everything possible to prevent recurrence. Others initially find it challenging to feel truly *finished* with cancer treatment when they continue taking medication.

What I want you to remember is this: maintenance therapy is not about living in fear of cancer. It is about taking proven steps to stay healthy.

The Bottom Line

Maintenance therapy represents one of the most significant advances in cancer care over the past two decades. These treatments have transformed outcomes for many patients, turning some cancers from fatal diseases into highly curable conditions.

When your oncologist recommends maintenance therapy, it is because the evidence shows it can significantly improve your chances of long-term survival and cure. While all medical decisions involve weighing benefits and risks, maintenance therapy recommendations are typically based on strong research showing meaningful benefit.

This is not about having more control over your care. This is about following the medical evidence that gives you the best chance of beating cancer for good.

So, as I began this chapter, the question of *How many more treatments, Doctor?* depends entirely on your treatment setting. Adjuvant and neoadjuvant therapies have predetermined endpoints based on clinical trial protocols. Metastatic disease typically requires ongoing treatment without a defined stopping point, although treatment breaks can sometimes be possible. Maintenance therapy, when recommended, is based on strong evidence showing improved outcomes for specific cancer types and situations. Understanding which category you fall into helps you know what to expect from your treatment plan.

Whether you have completed your treatment or are continuing with ongoing therapy, monitoring and surveillance remain critical parts of your care. The next chapter will cover the tools and schedules your oncologist uses to watch for any changes in your condition.

Part IV

Moving Forward—Reclaiming Your Health and Your Future

Chapter 14

After Treatment: The Surveillance Plan That Protects Your Future

Monitoring for cancer recurrence or progression is an important part of your care, whether you have completed your cancer treatment or are continuing with ongoing therapy. This chapter covers the various tools that oncologists use to track your progress and watch for any changes. We will discuss the timing and purpose of different scans, help you understand tumor markers, and explain newer technologies like ctDNA testing. Each monitoring method serves a specific role in your follow-up care. Our goal is to detect any problems as early as possible and when they are most treatable.

The Timing of Scans

Radiology scans are obviously a very important part of cancer care, providing crucial information at various stages of treatment. These imaging studies help in diagnosis, treatment planning, monitoring response, and assessing for recurrence. Here, we will discuss the timing and rationale for radiology scans pre-treatment, during treatment, and post-treatment.

Pre-Treatment Scans are often given before any treatment or surgery in order to help confirm the diagnosis and stage of the cancer. This is important for effective treatment planning and will often include either a CT scan, PET scan, or MRI, as discussed in Chapter 4.

During Treatment Scans are performed to monitor how well your treatment is working. The timing of these scans varies depending on your specific treatment plan, but they are typically done every three to four cycles during treatment. These scans help your oncologist determine whether the treatment is shrinking the tumor, keeping it stable, or whether adjustments need to be made to your therapy.

During treatment, we are looking for what we call a *response to therapy*. If scans show the tumor is getting smaller, that is excellent news, and we usually continue with the same treatment plan. If the tumor remains the same size, that can also be good news because it means the treatment is controlling the cancer. However, if scans show the tumor is growing despite treatment, your oncologist will probably recommend changing to a different approach.

Post-Treatment *New Baseline* Scans are performed after you complete your initial treatment to establish your new normal and to ensure that there is no detectable cancer. These scans serve as a reference point for future comparisons during your surveillance period. The timing of this baseline scan varies, but it is typically done one to three months after completing treatment, once any inflammation from therapy has settled down.

Surveillance Scans are the ongoing imaging studies done during your follow-up care to watch for any signs that cancer might be returning. The frequency and type of these scans depend on your cancer type, stage, and individual risk factors. Some patients may need scans every three to six months initially, then less frequently over time. Others may need imaging only if symptoms develop or other tests suggest a problem.

WORKBOOK CHECKPOINT: Before your next scan, use workbook page 14/1, **Scan Prep and Results Notes** to capture the scan details, prep instructions, and your top questions. Then use the same page to document the results and next steps. There is even a section on how to control scanxiety, page 14/4 **Five Micro-Habits for Scan Day**, for simple, repeatable tools you can use in the days leading up to the scan, the day of, and during the wait.

It is important to understand that the goal of scanning changes throughout your cancer journey. Before treatment, we scan to plan your care. During treatment, we scan to see if the therapy is working. After treatment, we scan to catch any problems early. Each scan serves a different purpose, and the timing is carefully planned based on when the information will be most useful for your care.

Surveillance Guidelines

Every cancer subtype has its own standard of care for surveillance once initial treatment has been completed. These guidelines are created by experts in the field of oncology for each cancer subtype through the National Comprehensive Cancer Network (NCCN). NCCN is a not-for-profit alliance of thirty-three leading cancer centers in the United States. The website includes an excellent section for patient education (www.nccn.org/patientresources/patient-resources).

Below, I have summarized some of the most important points regarding cancer surveillance from the accepted national guidelines. This is meant to give you a general overview, but it is by no means meant to replace the recommendations made by your oncologist.

WORKBOOK CHECKPOINT: For a quick, printable snapshot of typical follow-up schedules, see workbook page 14/2: **Surveillance Guidelines (Typical Schedules).** Use it as a reference point when you're scheduling visits and tests, and then compare it to the individualized plan your oncologist recommends.

Breast Cancer Surveillance

After initial treatment, my follow-up schedule typically includes a history and physical exam every three to six months for the first three years, then every six to twelve months for years four to five, and annually after year five. Imaging generally includes annual mammography, with breast MRI when clinically indicated. Routine lab tests (including tumor markers) are not recommended for standard surveillance, although many physicians will continue to draw them. Longer-term priorities commonly include bone health, heart health, and monitoring for treatment complications such as lymphedema. Additionally, lifestyle factors that support recovery should include a discussion of menopause symptoms, regular exercise, and a healthy, balanced diet.

Ovarian Cancer Surveillance

After treatment, my usual schedule for follow-up visits is typically more frequent early on: every two to four months for the first two years, then every three to six months for years three to five, and annually after year five. Imaging is not done on a fixed schedule; instead, it is generally performed when symptoms arise or when there is a significant change in the CA-125 protein (if CA-125 is being used). Lab monitoring may include CA-125 only if it was elevated at baseline and has proven useful for that individual patient's surveillance. Broader considerations often include genetic counseling/testing, if not already done, monitoring for longer-term treatment effects, and attention to bone health, heart health, menopause symptoms, and weight management over time.

Endometrial Cancer Surveillance

My typical follow-up includes a history and physical exam every three to six months for the first two years, then every six to twelve months for years three to five, and annually after year five. Imaging is generally symptom-driven (or based on exam findings) rather than routine. Routine lab testing is not recommended, although in some cases a provider may advise a vaginal cuff smear. Longer-term priorities commonly include bone health and lifestyle adjustments, as with breast and ovarian cancer, in an effort to support recovery and overall wellness.

Tumor Markers

The use of tumor markers in cancer care usually refers to the measurement of a specific protein level in the blood that is released by cancer cells. Common blood tumor markers in women's cancers include CA27-29, CA15-3, and sometimes CEA in breast cancers, CA125 in ovarian cancers, CA19-9 in pancreatic cancers, and CEA in colorectal cancers. The blood level of the tumor marker should be measured prior to treatment or surgery for a baseline and is later used as a reference. The marker is expected to decline following surgery, chemotherapy, or other treatment for the cancer. If it does not decline, or if it declines but not at the expected rate or amount, then it is often an indicator that the cancer may be growing and potentially is resistant to the current treatment.

It is important to note that tumor markers are not always reliable or representative of the volume of cancer present. There are several scenarios where this may be the case.

Non-Specific Elevations

Sometimes, tumor markers are elevated for non-cancerous conditions. A classic example is in ovarian cancer. CA125 can be elevated in ovarian cancer but also in benign conditions like endometriosis, pelvic inflammatory disease, and even during menstruation. CEA, a marker used in colorectal cancer, can also be seen elevated in patients who smoke or who have inflammatory bowel disease. An elevated marker may also persist after cancer surgery. Post-surgery or even radiation, there can be inflammation in the area of the cancer that may cause elevated tumor marker levels. These elevations are usually short-lived and progressively go down on their own post-procedure.

Early-Stage Cancer

Some tumor markers, such as CA125, CEA, and CA15-3, are rarely elevated in the early stages of ovarian, colorectal, or breast cancer, respectively. This is why sending tumor markers is not used as a screening tool to detect early cancers.

Tumor Variability

Not every cancer makes the proteins measured as tumor markers, and some cancers make more than others. This is one reason why patients should not *compare* tumor marker levels. I have had patients with elevated markers and no evidence of disease on scans, while another patient has a normal marker level but has extensive cancer—this is particularly common in some ovarian cancers. It is not uncommon for tumors to contain some cells that make the tumor marker protein and some that do not. This is called tumor heterogeneity and means that the tumors may consist of different cells that are related but may not be the same. Tumor heterogeneity may exist within a single focus of a single tumor or may differ among separate tumors.

Change in Production

Another important scenario is that the tumor marker production by the cancer cells may change with time and treatment. It is possible for the tumor to evolve and change when exposed to chemotherapy, but not be killed. Some cells may mutate to a form that no longer produces the tumor marker protein. These cells that no longer produce the protein may also acquire resistance to treatment as well, as they continue to evolve.

A last word about tumor markers. In my experience, patients and their loved ones feel obligated to track their markers. Some go as far as plotting on a spreadsheet and a graph. Although I understand and empathize with this practice, I want to leave you with a word of caution again. Tumor markers have limitations and are not the final word on cancer treatment success or failure. As discussed above, there are many reasons why tumor markers may vary, so please be cautious before jumping to conclusions, regardless of which way the marker is fluctuating. Traditionally, radiology scans are the best way for your oncologist to measure a response to treatments.

That said, the landscape of cancer monitoring continues to evolve. While we rely on proven methods like imaging and traditional tumor markers, advances in DNA technology have introduced another monitoring approach that oncologists are beginning to use: ctDNA monitoring.

Monitoring with ctDNA: A New Tool in Your Follow-up Care

You learned about ctDNA testing in Chapter 5, where we discussed its current limitations for initial diagnosis and early detection. But there are currently two areas where ctDNA is showing real promise and is increasingly being used in clinical practice: monitoring patients who have already been treated for cancer and patients who are living with cancer long term.

The key to making ctDNA less confusing is understanding that it means something different depending on where you are in your cancer journey. Are you still on adjuvant treatment after surgery, trying to prevent recurrence? Are you finished with all active treatment and now in surveillance? Or are you living with metastatic or recurrent disease? What your oncologist is looking for, and what a result means, is different in each situation.

How ctDNA Monitoring Works

Think of ctDNA monitoring like a very sensitive smoke detector. Just as a smoke detector can alert you to a fire before you can see flames, ctDNA can sometimes detect cancer activity before it shows up on scans or causes symptoms.

After treatment, if no cancer cells are actively growing and dividing, there should be little to no tumor DNA circulating in your blood. If cancer starts to return, those cells may begin shedding DNA fragments back into your bloodstream. ctDNA tests can sometimes pick up this activity weeks or even months before a tumor becomes large enough to appear on imaging. Whether knowing earlier actually changes long-term outcomes is still being studied, and the answer may be different depending on your cancer type and treatment situation.

If You Are Still on Adjuvant Treatment

Adjuvant treatment means you have had surgery and are now receiving additional therapy, such as chemotherapy, radiation, hormone therapy, or targeted therapy, to reduce the risk of the cancer coming back. In this setting, ctDNA is being studied to measure whether treatment is working at a molecular level and whether the dose or type of treatment should be adjusted.

Here is what the research is currently showing. In certain breast cancer subtypes, studies have found that ctDNA status during or after adjuvant therapy can be a stronger signal of recurrence risk than whether or not visible cancer remained at surgery. Women whose ctDNA was undetectable had very high rates of remaining disease-free at five years. Women with detectable ctDNA faced a substantially higher risk of recurrence (Hunter et al. 2026). These findings suggest that ctDNA may be measuring something that pathology alone cannot.

But here is the distinction your oncologist will want you to understand: ctDNA is currently a powerful signal, but it is not yet a proven instruction. No clinical trial has yet shown that changing your adjuvant treatment based on a positive ctDNA result improves outcomes. And no trial has shown it is safe to stop adjuvant therapy early based on a negative result. The research is actively underway, and this guidance may change. For now, a positive ctDNA result while your scans are clear is best addressed through enrollment in a clinical trial designed to study exactly this situation, or through continued close monitoring with your team (Kahl 2026).

If You Have Finished Treatment and Are in Surveillance

Surveillance means you have completed all active treatment and are now in a follow-up phase, typically with periodic imaging, lab work, and clinical visits. In this setting, ctDNA is being studied as an early warning tool for recurrence, the idea being that a rising ctDNA might signal that cancer is returning before it becomes visible on a scan.

The same caution applies here. A positive ctDNA result while your scans remain clear is not yet an automatic trigger for treatment. Guidelines from major oncology organizations acknowledge ctDNA as a supplemental tool, particularly when tissue biopsy is not possible, but do not yet support using it alone to make major treatment decisions (McKay et al. 2026). If your oncologist orders ctDNA during surveillance and it comes back positive, the next step is typically a staging scan to look for visible disease, followed by a conversation about whether a clinical trial might be appropriate.

In both the adjuvant and surveillance settings, a negative ctDNA result is reassuring but does not replace your standard follow-up schedule. Some cancers are low shedders that do not release much DNA into the bloodstream. ctDNA does not replace your scans, labs, and clinical visits.

If You Are Living with Metastatic or Recurrent Disease

This is where ctDNA has the most established role in clinical practice. If you are receiving ongoing treatment for metastatic disease, ctDNA can be used in two practical ways: tracking whether treatment is working, and identifying mutations that explain why a therapy may have stopped working.

Tracking Response Trends

Falling ctDNA levels often indicate that treatment is effective. Rising levels may suggest it is time to consider a change. Your oncologist will always look at ctDNA alongside your symptoms, exam, and imaging before making any decisions.

Identifying New Mutations

This is often also called a liquid biopsy. It is a blood-based way to look at tumor-related DNA without needing a new tissue biopsy, which is especially helpful when a repeat biopsy would be difficult or risky. In certain breast cancers, ctDNA can identify specific mutations that explain why a therapy stopped working and point toward what to try next. For example, in ER-positive tumors, a mutation called ESR1 can develop under treatment pressure and signal that a change in therapy is needed (Bidard et al. 2022), (Parsons et al. 2026). This use of ctDNA is already part of standard care.

What the Results Mean

Rising levels can be an early signal that cancer may be returning or progressing. But a rise does not automatically mean the cancer is growing. Effective treatment can cause many cells to die at once, temporarily releasing more DNA. Surgery and normal healing release DNA. Infections, inflammation, and even normal aging can create background noise. This is why oncologists interpret a rising result in context, often repeating the test before making major changes.

Falling or undetectable levels are generally reassuring. But a negative ctDNA test is not a guarantee. Some cancers are low shedders that do not release much DNA into the bloodstream, so a negative result does not equal a clean bill of health.

Stable levels over time typically suggest that treatment is controlling the disease, or that the cancer remains undetectable.

Patient Spotlight: Jane

Jane is a fifty-six-year-old woman who had Stage II ER+ breast cancer and received adjuvant chemotherapy followed by letrozole and ribociclib. The plan was for at least five years of therapy. She was tolerating the treatment fairly well until about two years later, when things started to shift. She started to have a lot of pain in her back and along her right rib. Her oncologist ordered a PET scan after her tumor markers were abnormal. Unfortunately, Jane's PET scan showed a few hypermetabolic (hot) spots in the bones, including her spine and her ribs. We opted for ctDNA testing instead of requiring another tissue biopsy, since it could give us information more quickly and without an invasive procedure. The ctDNA result showed a new ESR1 mutation. That finding helped us in two ways. It helped explain why the letrozole plus ribociclib was no longer controlling the cancer, because the cancer had returned and had evolved under treatment pressure. This result also helped guide the next line of therapy because now we were not guessing. We were making a decision based on how the tumor's biology had changed.

The Bottom Line

Monitoring ctDNA represents a genuinely exciting advance. It can tell us things about what is happening inside your body that scans alone cannot. In the metastatic setting, it is already an established part of care. In the adjuvant and surveillance settings, the science is maturing rapidly, and clinical trials are actively working to answer the question of what to actually do with the information once we have it.

For now, think of ctDNA as one instrument in a larger orchestra. Scans, tumor markers, physical exams, and ctDNA each contribute something different. None of them plays the whole piece alone. And the conductor, your oncologist, is the one who knows how to read the full score.

WORKBOOK CHECKPOINT: If your oncologist orders ctDNA, use workbook page 14/3, **My ctDNA/Liquid Biopsy Tracking Log,** to record the date, purpose, result (detected versus not detected), mutations, if any, and what action your team took. This prevents results from feeling like random numbers and helps you see trends over time.

Therefore, ctDNA monitoring represents an exciting advance in cancer care, offering the potential for earlier detection of recurrence and more personalized follow-up plans. However, it's not right for every patient or every situation. Currently, effective cancer surveillance involves multiple tools working together. Scans monitor for visible disease, tumor markers track protein levels, and newer technologies like ctDNA testing may detect microscopic changes earlier. Each cancer type has established surveillance protocols based on research showing what works best for detecting recurrence, though many will need to be updated soon since surveillance approaches continue to evolve as we learn more about what works best for detecting different types of cancer.

WORKBOOK CHECKPOINT: Your follow-up plan is not *one-size-fits-all.* Different cancers use different scans and different blood markers. Tracking the right items helps you and your oncology team spot meaningful change early (and avoid unnecessary worry from tests that don't apply to you). Use worksheet page 14/2 **Master Sheet for Surveillance and Tracking** to build your personal surveillance dashboard and keep everything in one place.

Chapter 15

Rebuilding Your Strength and Finding Your Footing: Moving Forward

As the final dose of chemotherapy settles into the rearview mirror, the journey through cancer treatment does not end; it simply enters a new phase. This chapter is designed to guide you through the often-overlooked challenges of the post-treatment landscape. Here, I review the physical, emotional, and psychological shifts that occur once active treatment concludes, and we introduce strategies to monitor your health, prevent recurrence, and nurture your recovery. My goal is that this chapter will help you navigate the complex terrain of life after cancer and can be used as a reference guide going forward.

Commonly Asked Questions

Over the years, I have noted that most patients ask the same, very practical questions after completing chemotherapy. I refer to them as the *When can I…?* questions, which usually include things like coloring hair, dental cleanings, exercise, eye exams, manicures or pedicures, and travel. The answer is often: *It depends.* Timing varies based on blood count recovery, infection risk, lingering side effects, and the specific treatments you received. I have summarized my general guidance in the workbook to guide your planning, but you should confirm anything time-sensitive with your own oncology team.

When Can I Color My Hair?

It's usually recommended to wait at least six weeks after completing chemotherapy before coloring your hair. This allows time for your hair to grow slightly longer, become more resilient, and for the skin on the scalp to be less irritated. Always do a patch test first to make sure you do not have an allergic reaction to the dye. I also usually recommend that in the first six months, you consider using gentle, ammonia-free dyes, which are less harsh on the newly sprouted hair.

When Can I Have My Teeth Cleaned?

Oral health is very important, especially after chemotherapy, which can adversely affect the health of your gums and teeth. Research shows that 28 percent of chemotherapy patients develop tooth decay, and about 20 percent experience severe gum disease (Hong et al. 2010). Chemotherapy can damage tooth enamel and reduce saliva production, creating an environment where harmful bacteria thrive. You can generally have your teeth cleaned once your white blood cell count returns to normal, and your oncologist confirms that your immune system has sufficiently recovered. This is often around a month after completing treatment, but the timing can vary based on individual recovery.

When Can I Start or Increase My Exercise?

Physical activity can be increased gradually as soon as you feel up to it, but check with your care team first if you have any restrictions related to surgery sites, port placement, or ongoing treatments. It's important to start slowly and increase the intensity based on how you feel. Activities like walking can be started fairly soon, and you can build up to more strenuous exercise as your strength and stamina improve. Consider adding weight training to your exercise routine, starting with low weights in the beginning. Patients will often lose muscle mass and tone during treatments due to lack of use, and it is great for your overall health and weight management to regain your muscles.

When Should I Get My Eyes Checked?

Chemotherapy can sometimes affect your vision, so it's a good idea to have an eye examination after treatment. However, I usually recommend that patients wait four to six weeks before undergoing testing because you can have mild swelling in the eyes that can alter vision from chemotherapy and the steroids, such as dexamethasone, which is used as a supportive medication. Please realize that this is a general recommendation for a patient completing standard chemotherapy. There are certain medications, such as some of the ADC drugs (antibody drug conjugates), which can cause specific eye changes that must be followed closely over a period of time.

When Can I Get a Manicure or Pedicure?

This is one of those questions that might seem trivial, but it speaks to getting back to the small joys that make you feel like yourself again. You should wait until your immune system has recovered and your blood counts have normalized, which is typically around four to six weeks after your last treatment. The concern here is infection risk. Manicures and pedicures involve cuticle manipulation, and even tiny cuts or nicks can become problematic when your immune system is still rebuilding. When you do go, choose a reputable salon that follows proper sterilization procedures. Better yet, consider bringing your own tools for the first few visits. And here is a practical tip: if your nails are still fragile or discolored from chemotherapy, a gentle buff and clear coat might be more comfortable than aggressive shaping or harsh polish removers.

When Can I Travel?

This depends on several factors, including your specific treatment, how you are tolerating it, and where you want to go. Some of my patients travel domestically to destinations with good medical facilities even during treatment, usually during their *off weeks* between chemotherapy cycles. The key is planning and communication. Before booking anything, check with your oncologist. We will consider your blood counts, energy levels, any lingering side effects, and the logistics of your destination. If you are planning to fly, keep in mind that air travel can be dehydrating and tiring, even under normal circumstances. For international travel, factor in your vaccination status, since some vaccines may need to be delayed after chemotherapy. Most patients can travel more freely about four weeks after completing their final treatment, but every situation is different. Start small if you can. A weekend getaway closer to home gives you a chance to see how you handle being away from your usual routines and medical support. Pack extra medications and bring copies of your recent lab results, just in case. The goal is not just to travel, but to enjoy it.

WORKBOOK CHECKPOINT: For a simple, printable guide to these "When can I…?" questions, see workbook page 15/1, **After Treatment: When Can I…? Quick Answers.**

Understanding the New Normal

As you transition from a structured world based around your treatment schedule to the rhythms of everyday life, it is helpful to understand what lies ahead. I have found that many of my patients have mixed emotions when completing treatment. Most, if not all, patients are happy to have completed active therapy, but many also have anxiety and fear. This is a complex jumble of emotions that may also include a sense of loss when they no longer have regular visits with their healthcare team. Patients have described feeling *safer* or *more protected* when seeing me more frequently during treatment, yet *alone* and even *abandoned* when they enter the surveillance phase.

If you have these feelings, you are not alone. This emotional whiplash is completely normal. But please realize that although you will not be seeing your healthcare providers as frequently, they are always, or should be, only a phone call away if something does not seem right.

What matters most is that you understand your specific situation and feel confident in your treatment plan. Some of you reading this may be dealing with ongoing treatment, while others may be done with active therapy. In either circumstance, make a commitment to yourself to live your best life.

I have also found that most of my patients continue to carry significant anxiety about their cancer returning. It is very important to understand your actual risk of recurrence because it is not the same across the board. Many patients will have what feels like an overwhelming level of fear about cancer recurrence that is not based on actual medical facts. That fear is real and valid, but understanding the facts can help keep it in perspective.

As you know, some forms of cancer have a higher risk of recurrence than others. Not all forms of breast cancer carry the same risk, and likewise, the risk of recurrence between different types of cancer, such as ovarian, uterine, colon, and breast cancer, is also different. As I reviewed earlier, the cancer stage, grade, cell type, and especially the cancer genetics are all important factors in whether a cancer recurs. It is very helpful to understand your personal risk of recurrence because this may help you cope better with your anxiety, especially if your risk is low. On the other hand, if you are at high risk of recurrence, you may choose to prioritize being more proactive in maximizing your best health and decreasing your risk of recurrence.

Oncology Follow-up and Surveillance

Cancer treatments, including surgery, chemotherapy, radiation, and targeted therapies, can have lasting effects on your body. Routine check-ups help manage these long-term side effects, which can include cardiovascular issues, hormonal imbalances, fatigue, and cognitive changes. By regularly consulting with your healthcare providers, you can address these issues promptly and maintain a better quality of life. But the caveat here is that you need to speak up. Do not suffer in silence with ongoing side effects such as hot flashes, vaginal dryness, or fatigue; make sure to tell your doctor so that we can help you. Please do not assume that this is a natural and expected aftereffect of cancer treatment that you must just endure.

Follow-ups should occur at regular intervals with your oncologist (surgeon and medical oncologists), your primary care physician, and possibly with your gynecologist if applicable. Often, in the case of gynecological cancers, the gynecological surgeon will take the place of a regular gynecologist while you are in active surveillance. In many academic medical centers, a cancer patient who is well may be transferred to a survivorship program for further surveillance after a couple of years. I know that many of my patients were initially unhappy about this, but in many respects, it is the best pathway. Often, surveillance clinics are run by nurse practitioners (NP) who are well trained in the standards of cancer surveillance, but they are also very in tune with general wellness care for women that the primary oncologist would not have necessarily had time to address. In my practice, the survivorship NPs would often converse with me about my patients and would absolutely refer them back to me if a new problem were to arise.

Risk of Recurrence

Even after successful treatment, there remains a risk that cancer could return. Regular follow-up appointments and screening allow your healthcare team to monitor for signs of recurrence. Early detection of a recurrence can lead to more effective treatment options and better outcomes. This ongoing vigilance is essential for maintaining peace of mind and health stability.

There is another important distinction to understand. In general, the risk of a cancer recurring for the first time is much less than if the cancer has already recurred before. The expected goal of adjuvant (preventative) treatment is to render you cancer-free and to prevent the cancer from ever returning again. On the other hand, when cancers recur, the goals shift. Treatment is usually focused on putting the cancer into remission (no evidence of disease), which is the best-case scenario, or keeping it stable and under control while maintaining your quality of life.

Risk of a Second Cancer and Routine Screening

Another important reason to stay on top of your healthcare and routine screening is that patients who have had cancer are at a higher risk of developing a second cancer, especially if there is a known genetic mutation. This does not mean it *will* happen, but it is important for you to be aware. Some cancer treatments can also increase this risk, and certain genetic factors that made you susceptible to your first cancer might put you at risk for others.

Fortunately, with routine screening and regular follow-ups, we will have the best chance of catching anything early, when treatment is most effective. These routine check-ups are not just about watching for a recurrence of your original cancer but also about staying vigilant for other potential health threats.

WORKBOOK CHECKPOINT: A printable summary of routine screening recommendations is in workbook 15/2: **Survivorship Screening and Routine Maintenance**. Use it as a reference, and then follow the individualized plan from your team.

Routine Healthcare Maintenance and General Wellness Care

For those of you who have finished treatment, it is important to talk about the medical care you will need going forward. Regular check-ups and screenings become your new normal, but the focus shifts from treating cancer to maintaining your overall health and well-being and staying vigilant for any changes.

Maintaining overall health is crucial for everyone, but especially for cancer survivors. Your cancer treatments may have affected other parts of your body in ways that are not always obvious at first. Some treatments, particularly certain chemotherapy agents, can affect the heart, bones, and hormone balance over time. Others can trigger or worsen conditions like high blood pressure, elevated cholesterol, or early menopause with its associated metabolic consequences. This is why receiving complete medical care is more important than ever, and why your oncologist and your primary care physician need to be in active communication with each other about your history and your ongoing needs.

Managing Chronic Conditions

Routine healthcare includes monitoring conditions like high blood pressure, diabetes, and high cholesterol, which may have already been present before your diagnosis, or may have developed or worsened as a result of your cancer treatments. Regular visits to your primary care physician help monitor your overall health, manage any chronic conditions, and address new symptoms or concerns that arise. Always keep your oncologist updated on these conditions as well. What happens in your primary care office matters to your cancer care, and vice versa.

Healthy Lifestyle and Dietary Habits

The American Cancer Society recommends a dietary pattern rich in vegetables, fruits, whole grains, and legumes, while limiting red and processed meats. The Mediterranean diet has shown particular promise for cancer survivors. A large Italian cohort study of 802 cancer survivors followed over nearly thirteen years found that high adherence to the Mediterranean diet was associated with a 32 percent lower risk of all-cause mortality compared to those who did not follow this dietary pattern, with an even more striking 60 percent reduction in cardiovascular mortality (Bonaccio et al. 2024). While I am certainly not a dietitian or nutritionist, what follows is what I have recommended to many patients based on my own education and innumerable referrals to nutrition specialists over the years.

So, what exactly is the Mediterranean diet? It is based on the traditional eating patterns of countries bordering the Mediterranean Sea. Think plenty of vegetables, fruits, whole grains, legumes, nuts, and olive oil as the primary fat source. Fish and poultry in moderate amounts, limited red meat, and minimal processed foods. It is not about restriction. It is about consuming an abundance of the right foods and avoiding the wrong ones.

Focus on eating a variety of colorful vegetables and fruits daily, aiming for five to nine servings. Choose whole grains over white or processed flour products, include plant-based proteins like beans and lentils, and limit red meat to no more than three portions per week. Avoid processed meats like bacon, hot dogs, and deli meats as much as possible. In 2015, the International Agency for Research on Cancer classified processed meats as Group 1 carcinogens, meaning the evidence that they cause cancer in humans, specifically colorectal cancer, is considered sufficient. This does not mean a single slice of deli turkey carries the same risk as smoking a cigarette. The classification reflects the strength of the scientific evidence, not an equivalence of risk. But for women who have already had cancer, this is a meaningful reason to make processed meats a rare exception rather than a regular habit (Bouvard et al. 2015).

Alcohol

This is a question I hear often, and the science has gotten clearer and harder to ignore. In January 2025, the US Surgeon General issued a formal advisory declaring alcohol the third leading preventable cause of cancer in the United States, after tobacco and obesity. The advisory identified a causal link between alcohol consumption and at least seven cancer types, including breast cancer, and noted that breast cancer risk begins to increase at consumption as low as one drink per day (Kwan et al. 2023). ASCO (American Society of Clinical Oncology) responded by endorsing the advisory and calling on oncologists to counsel their patients about alcohol as a behavior that increases cancer risk and one that we can actually control (American Cancer Society 2025). The World Health Organization and the International Agency for Research on Cancer have both stated plainly that there is no level of alcohol consumption that is without risk (World Health Organization 2023), (International Agency for Research on Cancer 2025).

When it comes to recurrence specifically, study results have not been entirely consistent. The largest studies suggest no significant overall association in the full population of survivors, though several found increased risk among postmenopausal women (Kwan et al. 2023), (Kwan et al. 2010). But those statistics do not tell the whole story. What we know about what alcohol actually does inside the body after a cancer diagnosis gives real cause for concern, regardless of what any single study shows. Alcohol works against you through several pathways at once. It raises estrogen levels in the blood, which feeds hormone-sensitive cancer cells. It breaks down in the body into a toxic byproduct called acetaldehyde, which damages DNA and blocks the repair systems that would normally catch and correct those errors. It triggers inflammation and generates unstable molecules that create an environment where cancer cells are more likely to survive and grow. And it depletes folate, a nutrient your cells need to copy DNA accurately. Laboratory studies have also shown that alcohol directly stimulates breast cancer cell growth and can blunt the effectiveness of hormone-blocking medications like tamoxifen and aromatase inhibitors (Kwan et al. 2010), (Kwan et al. 2013). That last point matters for anyone on endocrine therapy, because you are taking that medication specifically to suppress estrogen activity, and alcohol works in the opposite direction. The inconsistency across recurrence studies most likely reflects the challenges of this kind of research: alcohol intake is notoriously hard to measure accurately, breast cancer is not one disease, and many studies did not follow women long enough to capture the full picture. The biological mechanisms are not in dispute. For those reasons, my recommendation does not change: limit alcohol as much as possible, and if you can eliminate it entirely, the evidence supports that as the lowest-risk choice.

This is not about adding guilt to an already complicated life. It is about giving you the most current, honest information so you can make the decision that is right for you.

Cannabis

A conversation about cannabis use should be happening in every oncology practice, but most patients are not bringing it up with their doctors. In fact, a recent study showed that only about one in five cancer patients discussed their cannabis use with any member of their healthcare team (Ellison et al. 2024). That gap concerns me because the data on cannabis and breast cancer has shifted in ways that matter for the decisions you are making right now.

Forty-two percent of breast cancer patients use cannabis at some point during their cancer journey, most commonly for nausea, pain, sleep disruption, and anxiety (Weiss et al. 2022). Those are real symptoms that deserve real solutions, and I understand the appeal of something that feels natural and within your control. The FDA has approved two synthetic cannabinoid-based medications for chemotherapy-induced nausea, so this is not fringe territory. The problem is that what you buy at a dispensary is not a controlled medication, and for someone with a cancer history, that difference matters.

In 2024, ASCO published its first formal clinical guidelines on cannabis use in adults with cancer, plainly acknowledging that use has substantially outpaced the available science (Braun et al. 2024). Here is what the science currently shows.

Cannabis may interfere with your treatment. One observational study following women with newly diagnosed metastatic breast cancer found that cannabis users saw disease progression at 3.4 months compared to 13.1 months in non-users, and survival of 6.4 months compared to 28.5 months (Johnson et al. 2025). This was a single observational study, not a randomized controlled trial, and larger studies are needed before firm conclusions can be drawn. The numbers are still too significant to set aside while we wait for those studies.

Part of the concern comes down to how cannabis is processed in your body. Cannabis is broken down by the same system in your liver that processes many breast cancer drugs, including tamoxifen, aromatase inhibitors, and several CDK4/6 inhibitors. That can make your medications work differently than your doctor intends, sometimes too much, sometimes not enough. A 2025 study identified 412 potential drug interactions in 313 cannabis users, with 12 percent classified as causing major issues (Worster, Hajjar, and Handley 2022). For patients receiving immunotherapy, the concern is different but equally important. Cannabis may quiet the immune system, which is the opposite of what immunotherapy is trying to do, and early data suggests that cannabis use during immunotherapy may be associated with worse outcomes (Taha et al. 2019).

New data also raises questions about breast cancer risk. A 2025 study compared breast cancer incidence trends in states that had and had not legalized cannabis between 2000 and 2019. Breast cancer in women ages twenty to thirty-four rose 26 percent in cannabis-legalizing states versus 13 percent in non-legalizing states over the same period. The strongest signal was toward triple-negative breast cancer, the most aggressive subtype (Johnson et al. 2025). This does not prove that cannabis causes breast cancer. But it is a signal worth taking seriously, particularly when it points to the subtype with the fewest treatment options.

You may have seen headlines about cannabis killing cancer cells in laboratory studies. Those findings are real, and they come almost entirely from cell cultures and animal models, not from studies in people. Currently, there are no clinical trials demonstrating that cannabis treats or cures breast cancer in humans (Dobovišek et al. 2024). A survey found that roughly half of breast cancer patients who use cannabis believe it may be treating their cancer (Weiss et al. 2022). That belief is understandable. It is not supported by clinical evidence at this time.

If you are using cannabis or considering it, please tell your oncologist. This is not about judgment. It is about safety. What you put into your body during and after cancer treatment can affect how your other medications work, and your team needs that information to take care of you well.

Natural and Treatment-Induced Menopause After Cancer

One issue that deserves far more attention in survivorship care is treatment-induced menopause. Natural menopause is often a gradual transition, giving your body years to adjust as hormone levels slowly decline. Cancer treatment creates something entirely different. Chemotherapy, ovarian suppression, surgery, and hormone-blocking therapies can cause estrogen levels to drop from normal to nearly zero in a matter of weeks. The result is hot flashes, night sweats, sleep disruption, joint pain, mood changes, and vaginal dryness that arrive suddenly and with an intensity that natural menopause rarely produces. Think of it this way: a natural menopause is like watching the sun set gradually over an evening, whereas a cancer-induced menopause is like someone turning off all the lights at once. A 2025 survey of nearly 1,200 breast cancer survivors found that 94 percent rated their menopausal symptoms as moderately severe or severe, and nearly 80 percent said those symptoms significantly affected their quality of life, relationships, and ability to work. Despite this, fewer than 70 percent had been offered any treatment at all (Glynne et al. 2025). These are not just inconveniences, but real medical issues that deserve medical attention.

Patient Spotlight: Elena

When my patient Elena turned forty-two, she finished chemotherapy for hormone-positive breast cancer, and everyone told her she should feel grateful. Her scans were clear. Her hair was growing back. Life, supposedly, was returning to normal.

But inside, she felt like a stranger in her own body.

Night sweats drenched the sheets so thoroughly that she started sleeping on towels. Her joints felt so stiff she could barely button her blouse in the morning. Intimacy with her husband, once a source of comfort and connection, had become something she avoided. When she mentioned it at her follow-up, the nurse smiled kindly and said, "Yeah, that's common. It's just menopause."

But this was not just menopause. This was cancer-induced menopause, sudden and extreme, and layered on top of trauma. And while everyone celebrated her survival, no one was talking about the reality of living in this new body. Unfortunately, Elena's story is not unusual; it is the norm. And it is exactly why this section exists.

If you are experiencing these symptoms, please speak up. Do not assume you have to endure them. There are effective, evidence-based approaches that can be tailored to your cancer history and your goals. The first step is to be specific about what you are experiencing and how often it is happening. What follows is a practical guide to the most common symptoms and what can actually help.

Hot Flashes and Night Sweats

Hot flashes affect up to 80 percent of women after breast cancer treatment (Johns et al. 2016). They are not just uncomfortable. They disrupt sleep, work, and quality of life in ways that compound over time.

Venlafaxine, a medication that works on serotonin and norepinephrine pathways in the brain, has been studied in multiple randomized controlled trials and shown to reduce hot flash frequency and severity significantly in breast cancer survivors (Loprinzi et al. 2000). Gabapentin, a medication more commonly known for nerve pain, has also been shown in a large randomized trial to reduce hot flashes meaningfully, particularly nighttime symptoms (Mao et al. 2015). Paroxetine, a low-dose antidepressant, is the only FDA-approved non-hormonal medication specifically indicated for hot flashes, but notably should not be used by patients taking tamoxifen (Bordeleau et al. 2010).

Two newer medications work by targeting the brain pathway that directly triggers hot flashes when estrogen drops. Fezolinetant (Veozah), approved in 2023, has shown significant reductions in hot flash frequency in clinical trials, though liver function monitoring is required (Lederman et al. 2023). Elinzanetant (Lynkuet), approved in October 2025, has shown significant reductions in hot flash frequency and severity, specifically in women with hormone receptor-positive breast cancer on endocrine therapy in a phase 3 trial, with benefits sustained regardless of the type of hormonal therapy used (Cardoso et al. 2025). Ask your oncologist which option fits best with your other medications and your situation.

Beyond medications, several non-drug approaches actually work. Cognitive-behavioral therapy designed specifically for hot flashes has been shown in randomized trials to reduce the frequency and distress by addressing how your brain responds to the sensation itself (Johns et al. 2016). Acupuncture has been shown in a randomized trial published in the *Journal of Clinical Oncology* to reduce hot flash frequency and severity comparably to medication, with fewer side effects (Mao et al. 2015). Slow, controlled breathing can also reduce hot flash intensity by calming the nervous system response that triggers them (Johns et al. 2016). Practical adjustments help too. Layered clothing, a cool bedroom, a small fan on your nightstand, cooling pillows, and avoiding alcohol and spicy foods before bed are not just folk wisdom. My patients tell me these make a real difference day to day.

Vaginal Dryness, Discomfort, and Sexual Health

This is perhaps the most under-discussed consequence of cancer treatment, yet it profoundly affects quality of life and relationships. Vaginal tissue thins and loses elasticity when estrogen drops, making intercourse painful and sometimes causing chronic discomfort and recurrent urinary symptoms even when you are not sexually active. This is a biological change, not a personal failing. Please do not suffer through it in silence.

Non-hormonal options are the right place to start. Vaginal moisturizers, such as Replens or similar products, restore moisture to vaginal tissue when used regularly, two to three times per week. These are not lubricants for intimacy. They are tissue treatments you use consistently to address the underlying dryness. Vaginal lubricants, whether water-based or silicone-based, are separate and are used during intimacy to reduce friction and discomfort.

Vaginal dilators are medical-grade tools that can gradually restore elasticity and reduce pain over time. Pelvic floor physical therapy, performed by a specialized physical therapist, addresses muscle tension, scar tissue from surgery or radiation, and coordination problems that contribute to pain. Both of these approaches are underutilized and can make a meaningful difference.

Changes in libido are also common after cancer treatment and are influenced by more than hormones alone. Fatigue, body image changes, fear of recurrence, and relationship dynamics all play a role. If this is affecting you, please bring it up with your team. Referral to a sexual health specialist or counselor who works specifically with cancer survivors is appropriate and available. These are medical conversations, not embarrassing extras.

Hormonal Options

In most cases, low-dose vaginal estrogen for localized symptoms can be considered and is viewed as safe for many breast and gynecologic cancer survivors. Guidelines from the North American Menopause Society support considering low-dose vaginal estrogen for severe genitourinary symptoms when non-hormonal options have not provided adequate relief, with minimal systemic absorption shown in multiple studies (Faubion et al. 2018). This should still be a shared decision with your oncology team, particularly for patients on aromatase inhibitors or with strongly hormone-driven disease.

Systemic hormone therapy for menopause symptoms is a more complex decision that goes beyond the scope of this book. The decision to use it should be made between you and your physician after carefully weighing your cancer history, symptom burden, and potential benefits.

One emerging option worth knowing about is Duavee, a combination of low-dose estrogen paired with a medication called bazedoxifene that blocks estrogen's effects in the breast and uterus while allowing it to have positive effects in the brain and bone. A recent clinical trial in women with DCIS found that CE/BZA significantly reduced breast tissue cell growth compared to placebo, without negative impact on quality of life (Kulkarni et al. 2025). It currently carries a contraindication for women with a history of breast cancer and is not yet approved for this population, but the science is evolving, so it is worth asking your oncologist about, especially if you have a history of LCIS, DCIS, or ADH. For women with BRCA1 or BRCA2 mutations who have undergone oophorectomy, a large matched prospective analysis found that menopausal hormone therapy was not associated with increased breast cancer risk, and estrogen-only formulations were associated with a significant reduction in risk (Kotsopoulos et al. 2025). This is an important finding for previvors and should be discussed as an option with your oncologist. What I want you to take from this section is that you have options, and the conversation is worth having.

Joint Pain

If you are on an aromatase inhibitor, joint stiffness and pain are among the most common reasons women consider stopping their medication. Up to 64 percent of women taking aromatase inhibitors experience joint pain significant enough to affect daily activities (Glynne S et al. 2025). I want to be direct with you about this: stopping a highly effective cancer medication because of joint pain should be your last option, not your first.

Exercise is the single most proven intervention for aromatase inhibitor-associated joint pain. A randomized controlled trial published in *Supportive Care in Cancer* found that supervised aerobic exercise significantly reduced joint pain compared to usual care (Bender et al. 2025). A separate trial showed that even a home-based walking program reduced moderate-to-severe joint pain in breast cancer survivors (Nyrop et al. 2017). Movement increases the fluid that lubricates your joints and reduces inflammation. Start gently and build gradually. Think of it as physical therapy for your whole body.

If the pain is severe, it is also worth asking your oncologist whether switching from one aromatase inhibitor to another is an option. Different medications in the same class can affect people differently, and a switch sometimes resolves the problem without sacrificing the treatment benefit.

Menopause symptoms also connect directly to long-term health. Loss of estrogen affects bone density, can influence cholesterol and cardiovascular risk over time, and can worsen fatigue and cognitive symptoms, especially when sleep is disrupted. That is why the sections that follow focus on protecting bone and heart health and addressing these symptoms early, before they become the new baseline.

Bone Health

One of the more overlooked aspects of cancer treatment is what it does to your bones. Treatments like chemotherapy and especially hormonal therapies can significantly affect bone density, but this rarely gets the attention it deserves during your active treatment phase.

As women, we have the time until menopause, whether natural or treatment-induced, to build bone while we still have enough estrogen. After menopause, it is a downhill slide unless we actively work to prevent it. Many cancer treatments force women into a post-menopausal state much earlier than nature intended, which means bone protection needs to become a priority sooner rather than something to think about later.

With menopause, or treatments like aromatase inhibitors or hormone-blocking therapies, your bones start losing density faster than they can rebuild it. Chemotherapy can also interfere with the cells responsible for building new bone tissue. The result is increased bone fragility and a higher fracture risk.

Monitoring Your Bone Health

Your oncologist or primary care physician should be ordering regular bone density tests, called DEXA scans, to monitor bone loss. These are typically performed every two years. If they have not mentioned this, bring it up at your next appointment. These scans are quick, painless, and give us valuable information about how your bones are holding up.

The test results will show your T-score. Here is how to understand it:

- Above -1.0: Normal bone density
- Between -1.0 and -2.5: Osteopenia (lower than normal, but not yet osteoporosis)
- Below -2.5: Osteoporosis (significant bone loss requiring more aggressive treatment)

Your Bone-Protecting Action Plan

Since we are now working against the clock of treatment-induced menopause, every intervention matters more.

Calcium and Vitamin D: The Dynamic Duo

The Bone Health and Osteoporosis Foundation recommends 1,200 mg of calcium daily for women over fifty, but your body can only absorb about 500 mg at a time, so spread it out over the day (Bone Health and Osteoporosis Foundation 2024). There are reports that taking all of your calcium through supplements is detrimental, and I would agree. I usually recommend getting roughly half through food and the other half through a supplement. Think dairy products, fortified plant milks, leafy greens, and canned fish with bones. Pair your calcium with vitamin D3 and K2, because calcium cannot do its job without them. Vitamin D3 in the range of 1,000-to-2,000 IU daily is a reasonable starting point, but the right dose depends on your blood level (Bone Health and Osteoporosis Foundation 2024).

Have your Vitamin D level checked, ordered as a Vitamin D 25-OH blood test, at least once. A level between 30-60 ng/mL is widely accepted as the target range, though some research and many clinicians argue that the higher end of that range, or even somewhat above it, may be more beneficial for overall metabolic health. This is worth discussing with your physician because the right target for you may depend on factors specific to your health history. If you prefer to skip the K2 supplement, remember that it is also found in vegetables like spinach, broccoli, and brussels sprouts. Eat your greens.

Weight-Bearing Exercise: Your Bones' Best Friend

Your bones need stress to stay strong, the good kind of stress that comes from weight-bearing exercise. Walking, dancing, strength training, and even gardening counts. Aim for thirty minutes of weight-bearing activity most days of the week. Swimming, while great for your heart and muscles, does not help your bones as much because the water supports your weight.

What About Bone-Building Medications?

If your bone density drops significantly, your doctor may recommend medications like bisphosphonates, which include Fosamax, Boniva, and intravenous zoledronic acid, or a newer treatment called denosumab (Prolia). These medications are highly effective at protecting bone density and reducing fracture risk. There is an important additional reason to take this conversation seriously. A large meta-analysis of individual patient data from nearly nineteen thousand women in randomized trials found that adjuvant bisphosphonates significantly reduced breast cancer recurrence in bone, overall distant recurrence, and breast cancer mortality in postmenopausal women (Early Breast Cancer Trialists' Collaborative Group 2015). This means that for women who are postmenopausal at the time of treatment, bone-protecting medications may also be doing anticancer work. This is a conversation worth having, specifically with your oncologist, not just your primary care physician.

The Lifestyle Factors That Matter

Limit or eliminate alcohol, since more than two drinks daily can interfere with bone formation. Avoid smoking, which accelerates bone loss. Be mindful of excess caffeine and salt, both of which can increase calcium loss from the body.

A Word About Falls

As we age, and especially during treatment, balance and strength can be affected. The best bones in the world will not help if you fall hard enough. Make sure your home is well-lit, remove tripping hazards, and consider a balance, yoga, Pilates, or tai chi class if you feel unsteady.

The bottom line is that protecting your bones is protecting your future independence and quality of life. And since treatment may have shortened your natural bone-building window, there is no time like the present to get serious about this.

Heart Health

Cancer treatments can have significant impacts on cardiovascular health, though this is another area that often gets overlooked during active treatment. Certain chemotherapy drugs, radiation therapy to the chest area, and some targeted therapies can affect your heart function both during and after treatment.

Which Treatments Affect Your Heart

Anthracycline chemotherapies, like doxorubicin (Adriamycin), are particularly known for their potential cardiac effects, which may be irreversible and are related to cumulative lifetime dose. This is one reason your oncologist tracks how much you have received over your lifetime. Trastuzumab (Herceptin) and other HER2-targeted therapies can also affect heart function, but these effects are usually reversible when the medication is stopped. Radiation to the chest area, whether for breast cancer, lung cancer, or lymphomas, can affect the heart muscle and blood vessels over time.

A specific word about radiation and your heart. Older studies showed that women who received left-sided breast radiation had significantly higher rates of coronary artery disease compared to those who received right-sided radiation, because more of the heart falls within the radiation field on the left side (Carlson et al. 2021). The good news is that modern radiation techniques, including breath-hold techniques that move the heart away from the treatment field, have substantially reduced this risk. A large population-based study published in 2026 found that contemporary radiation methods are now associated with only minimal increases in long-term cardiovascular risk (Nakajima et al. 2026). If you received left-sided chest radiation, particularly before 2010, make sure your cardiologist or primary care physician knows this when evaluating your heart health going forward.

Monitoring Your Heart Health

Your oncology team should have ordered baseline heart function tests before starting cardiotoxic treatments, typically an echocardiogram or MUGA scan, with follow-up during and after treatment if you received heart-affecting therapies (Armenian et al. 2017). More comprehensive cardiovascular evaluation, including cholesterol screening and blood pressure monitoring, is typically handled by your primary care physician or cardiologist. Menopause can also shift cardiovascular risk over time, which is another reason to keep routine primary care visits and blood work on schedule.

If you notice symptoms like unusual shortness of breath, chest pain, or significant fatigue, do not dismiss these as just treatment side effects. Bring them to your team promptly.

Protecting Your Heart

Much heart disease is preventable through the same choices that support your overall recovery. Regular exercise, even gentle walking, a diet rich in fruits and vegetables, limiting processed foods and sodium, maintaining a healthy weight, managing stress, and prioritizing sleep all matter. Work with your primary care physician to keep track of your blood pressure, cholesterol levels, and blood sugar. In postmenopausal women who have had breast cancer treatment, cardiovascular disease is now a leading cause of long-term mortality, which means your heart deserves the same vigilance you bring to your cancer surveillance (Armenian et al. 2017). Do not skip those routine appointments.

The Emotional Toll of Cancer Treatment: Understanding and Managing Lingering Effects

Cancer and its treatments can have lasting effects that extend well beyond the end of active treatment. The emotional and psychological impacts often persist long after the physical treatment concludes. In fact, some patients actually develop more anxiety after completing treatment than during it, because the structure of regular appointments and a clear plan disappears. Patients tell me they felt safer when they were actively being treated and seeing their team frequently. That feeling makes complete sense. And it is one reason why the emotional side of survivorship deserves as much attention as the physical.

Common Emotional Symptoms Post-Treatment

Anxiety

Ongoing anxiety about recurrence or the uncertainties of life after cancer is one of the most common things I see. It can be triggered by follow-up appointments, scans, or even unrelated health issues that suddenly feel threatening.

Depression

Feelings of sadness, hopelessness, or loss of interest in things that once brought joy are common. Depressive symptoms can arise from the physical and emotional exhaustion of the cancer journey, changes in body image, or the loss of a sense of normalcy.

Post-Traumatic Stress Disorder

PTSD is more common in cancer survivors than many people realize. Flashbacks, nightmares, and severe anxiety related to the cancer experience can develop, particularly in those who had intensive treatments or life-threatening complications. If these symptoms sound familiar, please bring them up with your doctor. PTSD is treatable.

Loneliness

Treatment ends, and the world moves on, even when you have not. Many survivors describe a sense of isolation or even abandonment once the appointments slow down. This is real, and it is not a sign of weakness.

Body Image

Physical changes from surgery, chemotherapy, or radiation can significantly affect self-esteem. Scars from ports or surgery, hair loss, and weight changes are common concerns. The disconnect between how you look and how you feel inside is something many survivors carry quietly. You do not have to.

Fatigue and Cognitive Changes

I wrote this section with a bit more detail because I think these are two of the most common symptoms I have seen in my practice. In addition, they have often not been explained well to patients.

Fatigue and cognitive changes, often called chemo brain, belong together because they are not separate problems. They share the same biological drivers, and they move together. On days when fatigue is highest, performance on cognitive tasks drops measurably, particularly in processing speed, complex attention, and the ability to hold multiple things in mind at once (Gullett et al. 2019). Treating one without addressing the other misses half the picture.

Cancer-related fatigue is not ordinary tiredness. It does not respond to rest in the way that normal exhaustion does. It sits at a deeper level, affecting energy, mood, and mental clarity simultaneously, and it can persist long after treatment ends.

Cognitive changes affect somewhere between 17 and 78 percent of breast cancer patients at some point during or after treatment (Demos-Davies, Lawrence, and Seelig 2024). They show up as difficulty concentrating, trouble finding words, slower processing speed, and a general sense of mental fog that is different from ordinary forgetfulness. One of the most important and least-discussed findings in this area is that these changes often begin before chemotherapy starts. The tumor itself, and the inflammatory response it triggers from the moment of diagnosis, begins affecting brain function early. Chemotherapy intensifies these effects but does not create them from scratch (Gullett et al. 2019).

Sleep disruption from hot flashes and night sweats worsens both fatigue and cognitive symptoms, which is another reason the menopausal symptoms discussed earlier in this chapter deserve medical attention rather than quiet endurance.

The encouraging news is that for most women, the most severe cognitive and fatigue symptoms are time-limited. Most women in longitudinal studies returned to near-baseline fatigue levels by twelve to twenty-four months after completing chemotherapy, and overall cognitive performance improved across the follow-up period (Gullett et al. 2019). The brain is resilient, and recovery is the norm. What the research tells us is to stop waiting passively for recovery and start actively supporting it.

Supporting Cognitive and Fatigue Recovery

Now that you understand what is driving these symptoms, here is what the evidence says you can actually do about them.

Both fatigue and cognitive symptoms are influenced by measurable physical factors that your care team can check. Anemia reduces the oxygen your brain receives and directly impairs memory and processing speed. Iron deficiency can do the same even before hemoglobin drops low enough to meet the clinical definition of anemia. Low albumin, which reflects nutritional status, affects neurotransmitter production. Vitamin D deficiency is independently associated with fatigue, depressive symptoms, and impaired cognition. Certain inflammatory proteins that are part of the tumor's own biology have also been identified as consistent predictors of cognitive impairment during and after treatment (Boschetti et al. 2025). These are trackable numbers. If you are struggling with fatigue or cognitive symptoms, it is worth asking your team whether your hemoglobin, ferritin, albumin, Vitamin D, and inflammatory markers (such as interleukin-6 and TNF-alpha) have been reviewed recently in the context of how your brain is functioning.

Diet and Nutrition for Brain Health

Diet matters for brain function. The MIND diet, which combines elements of the Mediterranean and DASH (Dietary Approaches to Stop Hypertension) diets and emphasizes leafy greens, berries, nuts, fish, legumes, and olive oil while limiting processed foods and red meat, has been directly associated with better global cognitive function in postmenopausal breast cancer survivors within one year of completing chemotherapy (Winschel et al. 2025). This is distinct from the general Mediterranean diet discussion earlier in this chapter. If you are struggling with cognitive symptoms, your diet is one of the most actionable places to start.

Omega-3 fatty acids, specifically DHA and EPA, have been associated with better cognitive performance in breast cancer survivors. Two fish meals per week, or one to two grams daily of combined DHA and EPA from a purified fish oil supplement, is a reasonable approach that is considered safe during and after treatment (Winschel et al. 2025).

Probiotics are worth considering. Chemotherapy disrupts the gut microbiome, and that disruption is increasingly understood as one pathway contributing to chemo brain. A randomized controlled trial in breast cancer patients showed that probiotic supplementation during chemotherapy significantly reduced chemotherapy-related cognitive impairment, and a 2025 meta-analysis confirmed cognitive benefits, particularly when continued for at least twelve weeks (Zhang et al. 2022). Multi-strain formulations are the most studied. These are widely available and low-risk.

Sleep

Sleep deserves to be treated as a medical priority, not a lifestyle preference. Sleep disruption carries the largest quality-of-life impact of any single symptom in breast cancer survivors (Huang et al. 2026). Practical steps include maintaining a consistent sleep and wake schedule seven days a week, keeping your bedroom cool and dark, avoiding caffeine after noon, and limiting screens in the hour before bed. If insomnia persists despite these measures, ask for a referral for cognitive-behavioral therapy for insomnia, known as CBT-I. This is a structured, evidence-based program that is the first-line treatment for chronic insomnia and is more effective long-term than sleep medication (Morin et al. 2004). It is distinct from general CBT and specifically targets the sleep disruption cycle.

Brain Training and Compensatory Strategies

Brain-training programs are digital exercises that target the specific cognitive domains most affected by treatment, including processing speed, working memory, and executive function. BrainHQ (brainhq.com) has the strongest evidence base in cancer survivor research, with published studies showing improvements in memory, executive function, and self-reported cognition in breast cancer patients (Oldacres et al. 2022). Sessions can be done from home on your own schedule.

Compensatory strategies are practical workarounds that reduce the daily burden of cognitive gaps while longer-term recovery continues. Using a written planner instead of relying on memory, breaking large tasks into written steps, scheduling cognitively demanding work during your highest-energy window, which for most people is mid-morning, and asking people to give you one piece of information at a time rather than a list are all evidence-based approaches that have immediate practical value (Oldacres et al. 2022).

How to Manage the Emotional Aftermath

Recovering emotionally from cancer treatment involves a blend of self-care, professional support, and community. Here are the approaches I recommend most often.

Professional counseling offers a safe environment to process emotions and develop coping strategies. Cognitive-behavioral therapy and other therapeutic modalities are particularly helpful, and many therapists specialize in working with cancer survivors (Gullett et al. 2019).

Support groups, whether in-person or online, provide a sense of community and understanding. Sharing experiences with others who have been through something similar can be remarkably validating. Most treatment facilities and hospitals offer their own cancer support groups, and many more are available through national organizations.

Regular physical activity has been shown consistently to improve mood, reduce fatigue, and enhance cognitive function in cancer survivors (Zhang et al. 2025), (Hung et al. 2025). Tailor your routine to your current capabilities and interests. Many cancer centers offer specialized exercise programs for survivors, and even a short daily walk is a meaningful place to start.

Medication may be necessary in some cases to manage depression, anxiety, or PTSD. This is not a last resort. It is a tool, and it is worth discussing with your physician or a mental health provider who understands your cancer history.

Integrative Medicine Techniques

Practices like mindfulness meditation, yoga, and deep breathing exercises can be genuinely effective at reducing anxiety and improving well-being, and they carry very little downside.

Mindfulness meditation involves focusing on the present moment without judgment, which helps quiet the mental noise that anxiety feeds on. Research shows it can lower anxiety and depression levels, improve mood, and enhance quality of life in cancer survivors (Boschetti et al. 2025). Several phone apps offer guided sessions specifically designed for cancer patients, with breathing exercises, body scans, and mindful movement that integrate easily into a daily routine.

Yoga combines physical postures, breathing techniques, and meditation. For cancer survivors, it can improve flexibility, strength, and balance while providing mental clarity and stress relief. Start slowly and build gradually. Many cancer centers and community organizations offer specialized classes, and online platforms make home practice accessible.

Deep breathing exercises are simple tools for managing stress and anxiety that you can use anywhere, anytime. Techniques like diaphragmatic breathing, 4-7-8 breathing, and box breathing work by slowing the nervous system response that drives anxiety. Start with a few minutes daily and build from there. Consistency matters more than duration.

Online Resources for Support and Information

If you are struggling, please do not do it alone. Many cancer survivors benefit from counseling, peer support, and trusted educational resources, especially during the transition out of active treatment.

> **WORKBOOK CHECKPOINT:** I have placed a curated list of survivorship support resources on workbook page 15/3, **Survivorship Support Resources**, so it is easy to find when you need it.

Conclusion

The emotional toll of cancer does not end when treatment does. For some, especially those living with advanced cancer, it continues indefinitely. Recognizing these symptoms, naming them, and asking for help is not a sign that something has gone wrong in your recovery. It is part of the recovery process. The goal is not to get back to who you were before. It is to build something sustainable going forward, with support, with honesty, and with the understanding that you have already done one of the hardest things a person can do.

Chapter 16

Protecting Your Future: The Environmental Risks You Can Actually Control

The Hidden Threat in Our Everyday Lives

With improving guidelines for survivorship, it is heartening to see that cancer survivors are becoming more focused on the critically important roles of a healthy diet, regular exercise, and medical follow-up. Nevertheless, I also felt it prudent to discuss the often-overlooked component of what may be contributing to our increasingly unhealthy population. Environmental toxins are likely to be one of the missing links in the development of many cancers, including those under the age of fifty, where the incidence is rising.

To be clear about the evidence: nothing in this chapter comes close to the cancer risk posed by smoking, heavy alcohol use, or asbestos exposure. But many everyday products in our homes and workplaces contain chemicals that can damage DNA or disrupt hormones, and the concern is less about any single product and more about the cumulative effect of these exposures used together across a lifetime. This rarely gets the attention it deserves during survivorship planning.

Once you have fought one battle against cancer, the last thing you want is to expose yourself unknowingly to substances that could undermine your recovery or increase your risk. The good news is that understanding these risks and making small, strategic changes can meaningfully reduce your exposure. You cannot control everything in your environment, but you can control much of what you bring into your home and put on your body.

Understanding the Two Main Threats

There are two main categories of environmental toxins that concern me most for cancer survivors: DNA-damaging agents and hormone disruptors.

1: DNA-Damaging Agents (Genotoxic Carcinogens)

DNA-damaging agents are chemicals that directly attack the genetic material in our cells, causing breakages or mutations that can lead to uncontrolled cell growth.

Some of the most common DNA-damaging agents we encounter in household products include formaldehyde, benzene, and other volatile organic compounds (VOCs). The International Agency for Research on Cancer has classified both formaldehyde and benzene as Group 1 carcinogens, the same category as tobacco and asbestos.

Protection from DNA-damaging agents is important to everyone, but even more so for cancer survivors and previvors who already have an increased genetic risk of cancer than the general population. Cancer treatments like chemotherapy and radiation can compromise your body's natural DNA repair systems. While these treatments target cancer cells, they can also affect healthy cells and their ability to fix DNA damage. In the case of previvors, this may mean that the cells in your body are already missing one of the naturally functioning genes that help repair damage. In either case, your body may be less equipped to handle additional toxic exposures than someone who has never had cancer.

2: Hormone Disruptors (Endocrine-Disrupting Chemicals)

Hormone disruptors, also called endocrine-disrupting chemicals or EDCs, work differently from DNA-damaging agents, but can be equally problematic.

Many of these chemicals act like fake hormones in your body. EDCs can also interfere with how cells divide and grow, cause epigenetic changes that turn cancer-promoting genes on or protective genes off, and have outsized effects when exposure occurs during critical developmental periods like pregnancy or puberty.

Four Ways That Endocrine Disruptors Can Cause Cancer

Mimicking and Blocking Hormones

Here's what happens—many of these chemicals act like fake or decoy hormones in your body. They can bind to hormone receptors and essentially trick your body into thinking it has more estrogen or other hormones than it really does. They can also block your natural hormones from doing their job. This is particularly problematic because it can stimulate the growth of hormone-dependent cancers like breast, prostate, and endometrial cancers.

Altering Hormone Production

These chemicals can interfere with your body's ability to make hormones properly and affect how your body breaks them down and gets rid of them. When your hormones get out of balance, it can promote cancer development.

Disrupting How Cells Behave

When these chemicals mimic or block your hormone receptors, they interfere with the normal signals that tell cells when to divide, when to grow, and when to die off naturally. This disruption can lead to mutations building up and cells growing out of control, which increases your risk of developing tumors.

Changing How Genes Work

This is a tricky concept called epigenetic change. This is where these chemicals can change how your genes behave without changing the genes themselves. Some of these chemicals can turn on cancer-promoting genes or turn off genes that normally protect against cancer.

The most common hormone disruptors include BPA, phthalates, parabens, and PFAS chemicals. They are in plastics, personal care products, cleaning supplies, and food packaging. What makes them particularly concerning is that they can cause biological effects even at low doses, and the effects accumulate over time. Here are some of the most common offenders.

The Specific Culprits in Your Home

Nonstick Cookware and PFAS Chemicals

One of the most significant sources of toxic exposure in many homes is nonstick cookware. The chemicals that give Teflon its non-stick properties, PFAS compounds, including PFOA and PFOS, are what scientists call *forever chemicals* because they do not break down naturally in the environment or in our bodies.

A large 2023 study of more than ten thousand adults from the National Health and Nutrition Examination Survey found that women with higher blood levels of certain PFAS compounds had approximately double the odds of a prior melanoma diagnosis, and there was also a link between PFAS exposure and prior uterine cancer diagnoses. The researchers noted that PFAS chemicals appear to disrupt hormone function in women, which is one potential mechanism for increasing the risk of hormone-related cancers (Cathey et al. 2023). PFOA was classified as a Group 1 human carcinogen by IARC in 2023 (IARC 2012), (IARC 2025).

PFAS chemicals are not just in non-stick pans. They are also used in stain-resistant fabrics, waterproof clothing, food packaging, and some cosmetics. They can be absorbed through the skin or leach into food, especially when heated.

My recommendation is to make the switch to safer cookware. Stainless steel, cast iron, and ceramic cookware do not contain these chemicals and can last a lifetime with proper care. I was not happy to give up my Teflon pans and had some difficulty relearning how to cook with them, so I feel your pain. Food may stick more initially, but with proper preheating and a little more oil or butter, good results are achievable without the toxic exposure.

Air Fresheners and Scented Products

Both plug-in and spray air fresheners release a cocktail of chemicals into your home's air that you then breathe continuously. Plug-in air fresheners release phthalates and volatile organic compounds. Spray air fresheners often contain formaldehyde and benzene (Dodson et al. 2012). What many people do not realize is that these chemicals do not disappear after you smell them. They settle on surfaces throughout your home, including countertops where you prepare food, and continue to off-gas for hours or days.

I would be embarrassed to tell you how many plug-ins I had to toss.

Safer alternatives include essential oils in a diffuser, simmering a pot of water with cinnamon sticks, cloves, orange slices, or rosemary, or simply opening windows. Certain houseplants, like spider plants and peace lilies, can also help naturally purify indoor air.

Scented Candles

Burning candles, especially paraffin wax candles with synthetic fragrances, releases benzene and formaldehyde into your home's air (Dodson et al. 2012). Paraffin wax is derived from petroleum, and when it burns alongside synthetic fragrances, the breakdown process creates these genotoxic compounds. The longer the burn time, the greater the accumulation in your indoor air. I love scented candles as much as anyone. I tossed around fifty of them.

Safer options include soy or beeswax candles with cotton wicks and no added fragrances, unscented candles, or battery-operated candles for ambiance without combustion products.

Body Products and Personal Care Items

We apply personal care products directly to the skin, which absorbs what we put on it. Many patients are surprised to learn about the chemicals commonly found in daily-use lotions, shampoos, and cosmetics.

Parabens are preservatives used in many personal care products that act as estrogen mimics in the body. Studies have detected parabens directly in human breast tissue, including in 99 percent of tissue samples from mastectomy patients, and higher concentrations have been found in malignant breast tumors compared to benign ones (Barr et al. 2012), (Downs et al. 2022).

Phthalates are used to help fragrances last longer and to make products feel smoother. They disrupt hormone balance and have been linked to hormone-related cancers. People who use fragranced body lotions and cosmetics regularly have significantly higher phthalate levels in their bodies. My own daughter fought me when I tried to get rid of these products, so be forewarned.

Many personal care products also contain formaldehyde or formaldehyde-releasing preservatives, which are direct DNA-damaging agents (IARC 2012), (IARC 2025).

The strategy I use for myself and recommend to patients is learning to read labels and making gradual switches. Look for products labeled paraben-free and phthalate-free. Avoid products that list fragrance as an ingredient, since this term often covers phthalates and other undisclosed chemicals. Choose products with fewer ingredients overall and consider fragrance-free options.

Plastic Food and Drinking Containers

BPA and its common replacement, BPS, are estrogen-mimicking chemicals that leach from plastic into food and drinks, especially when heated. If you have switched to BPA-free plastics thinking you solved the problem, I want to flag something important: BPS, the most common BPA replacement, has been shown in multiple studies to have similar estrogenic activity to BPA, and a 2022 study published in the *Proceedings of the National Academy of Sciences* found that BPS disrupted normal human mammary tissue architecture at low doses (Winkler et al. 2022). BPA-free does not mean safe.

The worst offenders are heated plastics, old or scratched containers, and plastics in contact with acidic foods like tomatoes or citrus. Microwaving food in plastic containers is one of the highest-exposure scenarios. Like most people, I ate many microwaved meals in plastic containers over the years and have been to a Tupperware party or two. Those all got tossed as well.

My recommendation is a gradual transition to glass containers for food storage and stainless-steel water bottles for beverages. Glass can go from the refrigerator to the microwave safely without leaching chemicals. If you must use plastic, never microwave food in it, avoid hot foods in plastic, and replace old or scratched containers. This also applies to plastic cooking utensils.

Cleaning Products

Household cleaning products represent a complex source of chemical exposure because we use multiple products throughout our homes, often in enclosed spaces with limited ventilation. Laundry detergents can contain formaldehyde and endocrine disruptors that may remain on clothing after washing, creating ongoing skin contact exposure. Floor cleaners and surface cleaners release VOCs (Volatile Organic Compounds) that linger in your home's air and settle on surfaces throughout your living space (Dodson et al. 2012).

The cumulative effect of these exposures is what concerns me most. While individual exposures might seem small, the combination of multiple cleaning products used regularly in enclosed spaces can create a significant toxic burden.

Simple alternatives such as white vinegar and baking soda handle most basic cleaning tasks safely and effectively, though I will admit I am not personally a fan of the scent. For patients who prefer commercial products, look for those certified by third-party organizations as safer alternatives. Start by replacing the products you use most frequently, since those represent your highest exposure risk.

Why This Matters for Cancer Survivors and Previvors

The Cumulative Effect

Environmental toxin exposure is cumulative. Small exposures add up over time, and multiple chemicals can interact with each other in ways that amplify their individual effects. There is a useful term for this: *body burden*. This is the total amount of toxic chemicals accumulated in your body over time from air pollution, food, personal care products, cleaning supplies, and countless other sources. While you cannot control all of these exposures, you can significantly influence many of them through the choices you make at home.

One patient of mine was shocked when she realized she was getting phthalate exposure from her air freshener, her lotion, and her laundry detergent, all at the same time. This is why addressing multiple sources of exposure is more protective than focusing on just one area.

Taking Control

This information is meant to empower you, not frighten you. These toxins have been in our environment for a long time, which is infuriating. But at least we know now, and we can make informed choices. You have already demonstrated extraordinary strength in dealing with cancer or a genetic predisposition to it. Managing your environmental exposures is simply one more way to take control of what you can. The science continues to evolve, and the principle remains consistent: reducing unnecessary chemical exposures is a reasonable, prudent, and increasingly well-supported approach to protecting your health. Every step you take toward reducing your toxic burden is a step toward a healthier future.

WORKBOOK CHECKPOINT: Ready to make this practical? Turn to workbook page 16/1, which is a summary table of the environmental toxins reviewed in this chapter. Pick one Priority 1 change and do it this week. Keep the table somewhere visible and let it guide your next swap when you are ready.

Chapter 17

The Truth About Supplements: Making Smart Decisions for Your Health

For the first time while writing this book, I hesitated before putting words on the page. The field of oncology operates on randomized, placebo-controlled clinical trials as its gold standard. When it comes to nutrition, supplements, and herbal remedies, that level of evidence is largely absent. These topics are barely covered in allopathic (conventional, evidence-based) medical schools. They are enormous subjects that can only be addressed at an introductory level here. And yet, they represent some of the most commonly asked questions in my practice. Every patient wants to know which supplements they can take.

I am going to do my best to answer that honestly, which means acknowledging what we know, what we do not know, and where the evidence is genuinely uncertain. My goal is not to dismiss supplements or to embrace them uncritically. It is to give you the most accurate picture I can, so you can make informed decisions with your oncology team.

The Supplement Landscape

The supplement industry operates under the Dietary Supplement Health and Education Act of 1994, which **does not** require manufacturers to prove their products are safe or effective before bringing them to market. The FDA can only intervene after harm has already occurred. The US dietary supplement market is currently estimated at over **sixty billion dollars annually** and growing (Office of Dietary Supplements, n.d.), (Grand View Research 2025). Walk into any health food store and you will find entire aisles dedicated to products claiming to boost immunity, fight cancer, or reduce treatment side effects. The internet and social media are saturated with supplements and the gurus who sell them. Cancer patients are often targeted with products promising hope and healing, and I understand the appeal completely. When you are facing cancer, you want to do everything possible to help yourself. Supplements feel like something you can control when so much else does not.

The reality is more complicated than the marketing suggests.

Patient Spotlight: Eva's Shopping Bag

When I first met Eva at her new patient visit to discuss treatment for her recurrent breast cancer, she mentioned in passing that she was taking a few supplements but could not recall all the names. She remembered magnesium and Vitamin D, along with something to help her immune system and another to energize her mitochondria. She promised to bring everything in for her next visit.

A week later, Eva arrived with a shopping bag full of supplement bottles and a detailed chart she used to keep track of them all. She admitted something that broke my heart: she had not told me about most of them initially because she was afraid that I would be mad or disapprove.

Eva's story illustrates three things I see repeatedly. First, patients often take far more supplements than they initially reveal. Second, fear of judgment prevents honest communication about what patients are actually doing to help themselves. Third, the desire to do something is so strong that patients invest significant time, money, and hope in supplements, even when the evidence is unclear.

I was not mad at Eva. I was grateful she trusted me enough to bring everything in. That shopping bag became the starting point for an honest conversation about what might help, what could hurt, and what was simply expensive but harmless.

Not all supplements are useless or dangerous. Some cancer patients develop genuine nutrient deficiencies due to reduced appetite, chemotherapy side effects, or the cancer itself. Blood tests can identify those deficiencies, and targeted supplementation can genuinely help. In my practice, the supplements I recommend in certain circumstances include Vitamin D3, omega-3 fatty acids, prebiotics and probiotics, magnesium, B-complex vitamins including B6, B12, and folic acid, turmeric, and iron.

I have intentionally not included specific subtypes or dosages here. Before starting any supplement, consult your oncology team to confirm it is safe, appropriate for your specific situation, and will not interfere with your treatment. Supplements should never replace your cancer treatment or a balanced diet. They are tools that can complement your care when used appropriately and under medical supervision.

When Supplements Become Dangerous: What You Must Know

This is the section I most need you to read carefully.

Patient Spotlight: Sarah

Sarah was receiving treatment for breast cancer when her liver function tests became abnormal. I stopped her treatment immediately, thinking the treatment itself was the cause. We waited several weeks. The tests did not improve. After weeks of worry and treatment delays, Sarah recalled that she had started taking new supplements a friend had recommended to help kill cancer and detox her liver. She had not put them on her medication list because she did not think of vitamins and supplements as medicine. When she stopped them, her liver tests returned to normal, and we were able to restart her treatment. Sarah almost missed getting the care she needed because of supplements she thought were harmless.

This is a true story from my practice, but unfortunately, not a rare one. Supplements can cause real medical problems that mimic treatment side effects, leading to unnecessary delays and worry. Please hear this clearly: ***natural* does not mean safe**. A wise mentor of mine once put it well: "Just because something is natural does not mean it is good for you. Tobacco and cyanide are both natural. Both can kill you."

Antioxidant supplements, including high doses of Vitamin C and Vitamin E, can potentially interfere with radiation therapy and some chemotherapy because those treatments work partly by creating oxidative stress to kill cancer cells. Large doses of antioxidants may reduce that effectiveness.

St. John's Wort deserves specific attention because it is one of the most commonly used herbal supplements and one of the most dangerous for cancer patients. It significantly speeds up how your liver metabolizes many medications by inducing the CYP3A4 enzyme system. In human clinical studies, St. John's Wort reduced blood levels of irinotecan, a commonly used chemotherapy drug, by approximately 40 percent (Mathijssen et al. 2002), (Mannel 2004). It can also significantly reduce blood levels of tamoxifen by the same mechanism, potentially undermining years of hormone therapy (Mathijssen et al. 2002), (Mannel 2004). This is not theoretical. It is a well-documented, clinically significant drug interaction that has led to treatment failures.

A third category of concern includes supplements that contain pharmaceutical-level compounds, are contaminated with unlisted ingredients, or are marketed specifically to cancer patients with claims they cannot support. Immune boosters, liver detoxifiers, and mitochondrial enhancers are common offenders. They are largely unregulated, often unstudied in cancer patients, and some carry real risks. Eva's shopping bag included three different immune boosters, two energy supplements, a liver detoxifying capsule, and a mitochondrial enhancer costing sixty dollars a month. None had clinical evidence for helping breast cancer patients, and one contained high-dose antioxidants that could have interfered with her upcoming chemotherapy.

Please tell your oncology team about every supplement, vitamin, and herb you are taking or considering. We are not here to judge you. We need to know in order to keep you safe.

A Word About Quality

If you do use any herbal supplement after discussing it with your team, please buy from reputable companies that conduct third-party testing. Look for seals from the United States Pharmacopeia or NSF International on the label. Studies have found that some supplements contain ingredients not listed on the label, including, in some cases, actual pharmaceutical estrogens added to make them appear to work. The label is not always an accurate guide to what is in the bottle.

Phytoestrogens: Separating Fear from Evidence

A significant category of supplements marketed to women with breast cancer involves phytoestrogens, plant compounds that weakly mimic estrogen. For years, women with breast cancer were told to avoid all phytoestrogens entirely. That blanket advice was based primarily on old rodent studies using extremely high doses. The human evidence tells a more nuanced story.

Before I review these individually, one framing point matters. Most of what follows involves laboratory studies using cell cultures or animal models. This type of research tells us about possible biological mechanisms, but it does not tell us what happens in actual human cancer patients. When human clinical data exist, I will say so. When they do not, I will say that too.

Soy and Soy Isoflavones

The most reassuring data in this entire section involves soy. A 2024 meta-analysis including over eleven thousand women and conducted in collaboration with researchers at Johns Hopkins found that soy isoflavones were associated with a 26 percent reduced risk of breast cancer recurrence, with the greatest benefit seen at sixty milligrams per day in postmenopausal women (van Die et al. 2024). The benefit was also seen specifically in estrogen receptor-positive survivors, which directly contradicts the older fear that soy was dangerous for hormone-sensitive cancers. Sixty milligrams of isoflavone is roughly equivalent to two to three servings per day of whole soy foods, such as a cup of soy milk, three ounces of tofu, or half a cup of cooked edamame.

The key distinction is whole soy foods versus concentrated supplements. Eating tofu, edamame, soy milk, and other whole soy foods appears to be safe and may be beneficial. Taking concentrated isoflavone supplements in doses far exceeding what you would get from food is a different matter and is not well studied during active treatment. My recommendation is to include moderate amounts of whole soy foods in your diet if you enjoy them, and to skip the soy supplements in pill form.

Flaxseed and Lignans

Flaxseed contains lignans, a type of phytoestrogen that has also raised concerns. The human evidence here is reassuring. Studies show that lignan consumption is associated with reduced breast cancer risk and possibly lower mortality rates. The American Institute for Cancer Research supports including one to four tablespoons of ground flaxseed per day as potentially beneficial for breast cancer survivors (Collins 2017).

The same food-versus-supplement distinction applies. Ground flaxseed added to oatmeal or a smoothie appears safe. High-dose concentrated lignan supplements are less studied and should be avoided until we have better evidence. If you are on tamoxifen, discuss flaxseed use with your oncologist first, as some monitoring may be warranted.

Black Cohosh

Black cohosh is one of the most studied herbal supplements in breast cancer patients. The current evidence does not support an association between black cohosh and an increased breast cancer risk. Multiple studies show it does not have estrogenic effects on breast tissue and does not appear to promote cancer growth (Fritz et al. 2013), (Castelo-Branco et al. 2021). This makes it less concerning than its reputation suggests.

The evidence for its effectiveness in treating hot flashes is, however, mixed. Some women find genuine relief. Others see no benefit. The interaction data with tamoxifen remains inconclusive, with some laboratory studies suggesting possible interference with efficacy and clinical studies not showing clear harm (Fritz et al. 2014), (Castelo-Branco et al. 2021). If you want to try black cohosh for menopausal symptoms, discuss it with your oncology team first. As I noted in Chapter 15, several prescription medications with stronger evidence are available for managing hot flashes.

The Gray Area Supplements

The supplements below have more complicated evidence profiles. What they share in common is that the data is largely preclinical, meaning cell culture and animal studies, with limited or no human clinical trials specifically in cancer patients. I present the current state of the evidence so you can have an informed conversation with your oncologist, not so you can make a solo decision on your own.

Dong Quai

This is used in traditional Chinese medicine for menopausal symptoms. A 2019 study found it was less stimulating to breast cancer cells than previously feared and challenged the blanket avoidance recommendation (Yue et al. 2019). Other studies show it can promote tumor growth in mice with ER-positive breast cancer. No clinical trials have looked specifically at dong quai in women with cancer. For women with ER-positive disease, caution is warranted. Discuss with your oncologist before using.

Red Clover

This contains isoflavones similar to soy but is typically used as a concentrated supplement. A three-year study of 401 women with a family history of breast cancer found red clover had no effect on breast density, uterine lining, or hormone levels (Powles et al. 2008). A 2013 review of 131 studies concluded that current evidence does not support breast cancer-promoting effects (Fritz et al. 2013). The data is more reassuring than the older guidance suggested. If considering it, then please discuss it with your oncologist first.

Ginseng

The evidence pulls in two directions simultaneously. A 2023 review found that ginsenosides, the active compounds in ginseng, show anti-cancer activity in laboratory and animal studies (Deng et al. 2023). However, some ginsenosides also act as weak estrogens in cell studies (Lee et al. 2003). The estrogenic versus anti-cancer effects appear to depend on which specific compounds are present and how the product was processed, which varies widely between commercial preparations. No way currently exists to predict reliably which effect will dominate in a given product. For women with ER-positive breast cancer, this unpredictability is reason enough to skip it until we have better clinical data.

Licorice Root

This contains compounds that go in opposite directions within the same plant. A 2023 Northwestern University study found that one compound in licorice, liquiritigenin, actually functions as an aromatase inhibitor (Hajirahimkhan et al. 2023), (Tamir et al. 2000). Other compounds in the same plant, particularly glycyrrhizin and glabridin, act like estrogen. Until researchers determine which preparations are safe and which are not, women with hormone-sensitive cancers should avoid licorice root supplements.

Chasteberry (Vitex)

Chasteberry works primarily through the dopamine system, affecting prolactin rather than directly mimicking estrogen, which initially seemed reassuring. However, laboratory studies show it can increase progesterone receptor expression in breast cancer cells and demonstrate some estrogen-like activity (Liu et al. 2001), (Jarry et al. 1994). We lack the clinical trials in breast cancer patients needed to make a confident recommendation. For hormone-sensitive breast cancer, skip this one until better data exists.

Evening Primrose Oil

This is the one supplement in this section with a clearly reassuring profile. Memorial Sloan Kettering Cancer Center states that evening primrose oil does not have intrinsic estrogenic properties (Memorial Sloan Kettering Cancer Center 2022). A 2022 study found it may actually enhance tamoxifen's effectiveness against breast cancer cells, and a 2023 study in patients undergoing chemotherapy found it reduced inflammation without safety concerns (Abd-Alhaseeb et al. 2022), (Arsic et al. 2023). It does not appear to act like estrogen and may be helpful. If you use it, buy a product containing only evening primrose oil without added herbs or compounds.

Wild Yam

Wild yam is frequently marketed as a natural source of progesterone or estrogen because it contains diosgenin, which can be converted into hormones in a laboratory but not in the human body. Any progesterone in a wild yam product was synthesized in a lab and added. Despite this, wild yams have estrogen-like effects. What wild yam actually does in the body is less clear, and the laboratory evidence is limited and mixed. One cell study found that wild yam extract had weak estrogen-like activity on some markers, yet in the same experiment it also lowered estrogen receptor levels and slowed the growth of breast cancer cells (Park et al. 2009). The hormonal signal is real enough to take seriously but too uncertain to call safe. For now, I recommend that you should not believe the "natural progesterone" marketing of this product, and for hormone-sensitive breast cancer, skip it.

The Bottom Line on Phytoestrogens

Dietary sources of phytoestrogens, particularly whole soy foods and ground flaxseed, appear safe and may be genuinely beneficial based on the strongest human evidence available. Concentrated supplement forms of the same compounds carry more uncertainty. The gray area supplements discussed above are not definitively dangerous for everyone, but none have been proven safe in clinical trials for breast cancer patients or others with hormone-sensitive tumors. When you are unsure, choose food over pills, and discuss any supplement with your oncologist before starting.

Conclusion: Navigating the Supplement Landscape

I need to be honest about my limitations here. I am not an herbalist, and I am not formally trained in alternative or functional medicine. What this chapter reflects is my personally attained knowledge and my experience caring for cancer patients over twenty-five years. I have done my best to review the available evidence, and I fully recognize that this world extends far beyond my training.

Opinions about supplements vary enormously, sometimes in polar opposite directions. You will find practitioners who prescribe elaborate supplement regimens for cancer patients. You will find others who dismiss them entirely. This lack of consensus reflects a genuine reality: we do not have the same level of rigorous, reproducible clinical evidence for most supplements that we have for conventional cancer treatments.

As an oncologist, my primary goal is to treat your cancer safely and effectively. Until more convincing evidence exists, many supplements are not supported.

Patient Spotlight: Eva

Eva and I spent fifteen minutes going through her shopping bag. We kept the magnesium and Vitamin D after checking her blood levels. We eliminated the immune boosters and the supplements that could interfere with her treatment. She saved money and reduced her pill burden, almost certainly without losing any real benefit. More importantly, she learned she could trust me with the whole truth about what she was doing for her health.

Patient Spotlight: Sarah

Sarah's liver recovered completely, and we were able to finish her treatment successfully. Her story has made me ask better questions of every patient I have seen since, especially focusing on asking them, "Please tell me ***everything*** *that you are taking or using."*

Please tell your oncology team about every supplement, vitamin, and herb you are taking or considering. We will not judge you. We want to keep you safe.

Epilogue

What I've Learned from the Bedside

Over my twenty-five years as a medical oncologist, I have been privileged to be part of thousands of women's most difficult conversations, which included raw fear, impossible decisions, devastating losses, and unexpected grace. My patients have been my greatest teachers, and as you close this book, I want to share what they've taught me and leave you with some final thoughts.

To all my patients, past and present: Thank you. This book is my attempt to honor what you taught me and to pass it forward to others who need it now.

What My Patients Taught Me

1. **Asking the right question matters more than having all the answers.** Early in my career, I'd ask patients, "How are you doing?" and take "Fine" at face value. I learned to pause, make eye contact, and ask, "How are you *really* doing?" That's when I'd hear about the insomnia, the panic attacks, the side effects they thought they just had to endure, the family conflicts they were navigating alone. The second question—the one asked with genuine presence—that's where the real doctoring begins.
2. **Every patient needs something different from me as their doctor.** Some wanted every detail: mechanism of action, clinical trial data, statistics broken down by subgroup. Others wanted the bottom line: "Just tell me what I need to do." Some needed me to be direct and matter-of-fact. Others needed more time to process emotions before discussing logistics. I learned to read the room, to adapt my style, to meet each person where they were rather than where I thought they should be.

3. **The hardest appointments aren't always about bad news.**
   Telling someone their cancer has progressed is devastating. But sometimes the hardest conversations are about finishing treatment, when patients feel terrified to leave the safety net of regular appointments and monitoring. Or when someone is cured but can't stop waiting for the other shoe to drop. And when a patient feels guilty for being exhausted by survivorship, when they "should just be grateful to be alive."

   And sometimes the hardest appointments are the ones where I know a patient is making a decision that will probably cost her life, but she doesn't believe me. I've sat with women who refused chemotherapy in favor of holistic treatments alone, despite extremely high-risk disease. I've explained the statistics, offered second opinions, tried every angle I could think of, and watched them walk out my door convinced that juicing, enemas, and supplements would be enough. Then, six months later, they're back with recurrent disease, and the window for a cure had closed. Those appointments haunt me. There's no protocol for watching someone you want to help choose a path you know is dangerous, respecting their autonomy while your heart is breaking.
4. **My job description extends far beyond chemotherapy.**
   I've spent hours on the phone fighting insurance companies that denied PET scans or genetic testing. I've written letters to employers about reasonable accommodations. I've connected patients with financial counselors, support groups, and mental health resources. I've helped families navigate end-of-life decisions with honesty and compassion. I've learned that being an oncologist means being an advocate, a translator, a coordinator, and sometimes simply a witness to suffering I cannot fix.
5. **People are capable of extraordinary adaptation.**
   I've watched women lose their hair, their fertility, their breasts, their sense of normalcy, and somehow find ways to keep living meaningful lives. Not because they're unusually heroic, but because humans are remarkably adaptive when they have no other choice. They didn't become *cancer*

warriors or *inspirations*. They just showed up, day after day, and did what needed to be done. That's real strength.

6. **To be honest about uncertainty.**
Patients don't need false optimism. They need truth delivered with compassion. When I don't know if a treatment will work, I say so. When the statistics are grim, but there's still reason to try, I acknowledge both. When someone asks, "How long do I have?" and I can't give a precise answer, I explain why. Honesty builds trust. Sugar-coating builds resentment. And no matter how many journal articles I read or conferences I attended, my patients regularly remind me that they are the experts on their own bodies and lives. The textbook doesn't account for the single mother who can't take time off work for weekly infusions. Or the patient whose quality of life on treatment is worse than the disease itself. Or the woman whose priorities shift when her grandchild is born. I have learned to create treatment plans with patients, not for them.

My Own Unexpected Turn

In 2024, my own health required me to step away from my very busy clinical practice. That decision broke my heart. For twenty-five years, my identity had been wrapped up in writing chemo orders, a packed schedule of patient appointments, and the privilege of being present in the most vulnerable moments of people's lives at a leading cancer hospital.

Leaving felt like losing myself.

But it also gave me something unexpected: time and perspective to write this book. For years, I'd wanted to create a comprehensive guide that could reach beyond my exam room—something that would translate complex oncology into plain language, provide organizational tools I knew made a difference, and empower patients to advocate for themselves.

I'm still doing what I've always done: listening, educating, organizing, fighting for patients. Just differently. Maybe more broadly than I could have in person, one appointment at a time.

This book is my way of continuing to serve and honor what my patients taught me.

What You Need to Hear (i.e., Your Takeaways)

As you move forward, here's what I need you to know:

You Don't Have to Have This Figured Out

Right now, you might feel like you're supposed to be strong, positive, and proactive. That's a lot of pressure. Here's the truth: some days you'll manage all of that. Other days you'll cry in the shower, snap at people you love, and feel completely overwhelmed. Both are normal. Give yourself permission to have hard days without judging yourself for them.

Bring Your Questions and an Advocate to Every Appointment

Write them down ahead of time because your mind will go blank in the exam room. No question is stupid. If you don't understand something, ask again. If your doctor seems rushed, say, "I need more time to understand this." If something doesn't feel right with your care, speak up. You're not being difficult—you're being an informed participant in your own treatment.

Build Your Support System Intentionally

You need a ride to chemotherapy. You need someone to take notes at appointments when your brain is too foggy to retain information. You need people who will bring you groceries, pick up your kids, or just sit with you when you don't want to be alone. Don't wait for people to offer—tell them specifically what would help. Most people want to do something; they just don't know what.

Use the Tools in This Book

The planner and binder aren't just busywork. They're how you create order in chaos. When you track your symptoms, your oncologist can adjust your medications more effectively. When you bring organized records, you save time and reduce errors. When you have your questions written down, you leave appointments feeling informed rather than confused. These tools work, but only if you use them.

Let Go of What You Can't Control

You can't control whether treatment works exactly as hoped. You can't control how your body responds. You can't control other people's reactions to your diagnosis. But you can control how prepared you are for appointments. You can control whether you ask for help. You can control whether you advocate for yourself. Focus your energy there.

Do Not Let Cancer Isolate You

Even surrounded by people who love you, you might feel like no one truly understands what you're going through. That's normal, and it's okay to acknowledge it. But here's what I want you to remember: you don't have to navigate this alone. You have a care team whose job is to guide you through every decision and every treatment. You have loved ones who want to help, even if they need you to tell them how. And you have resources—support groups, counselors, patient navigators—specifically designed to walk this path with you. Reaching out isn't weakness; it's wisdom. Let people help you carry this burden.

A Final Thought

Cancer changes everyone it touches. You won't be the same person on the other side of this that you were before the diagnosis. That's not good or bad; it just is.

But cancer doesn't have to define your entire existence. You're still you: complex, capable, worthy of excellent care and deep respect. You're still someone's daughter, mother, sister, friend. You're still someone with interests, opinions, and a life beyond doctor's appointments and scan results.

This book has walked you through the medical landscape of cancer: from diagnosis through treatment, monitoring, and survivorship. But the most important things I want to share with you are these:

- You have a voice. Use it.
- You have a care team. Hold them accountable.
- You have tools. Put them to work.
- You have people who love you. Let them help.
- And you have more strength than you probably believe right now. You'll discover it when you need it.

I've been honored to guide you through these pages. Though we may never meet, please know I'm rooting for you.

Go forward with clarity, with courage, and with the knowledge that you are stronger than you know.

Tiffany Troso-Sandoval, MD

Acknowledgments

This book is the result of three intersecting sources: the patients who entrusted me with their care, the friends who sustained my spirit, and the family who made it all possible.

To my patients: You have been my greatest teachers. You taught me what is truly important from your perspective and how to better communicate in moments that matter most. You showed me how to be a good doctor by reminding me that treating the whole person is just as important as fighting the cancer. Every page of this book carries the lessons you generously shared through your courage, your questions, and your trust.

To my friends: You gave me perspective on life outside of being a doctor. You taught me how to honor and respect one another, and how to laugh even when things get tough. Your encouragement and your ability to remind me that I am more than my white coat gave me the confidence to believe this book mattered.

To my family: Your unconditional love and our support for one another are the foundation of everything I am and everything I do. Luke, Tyler, and Gabriella, you are my shining stars and the center of my universe. Stuardo, you are my sun, my warmth, the source of light and strength that sustains me when everything else feels cold and impossible. To my mom in heaven and my dad, your unwavering support and belief in me gave me the courage to pursue this calling and the resilience to see it through. You are *all* the reason I have the strength to give so much to my patients and my work. This book exists because you believed in me, even when I doubted myself.

Endnotes

Abd-Alhaseeb, Mohammad M., Sarah M. Massoud, Fatma Elsayed, Gamal A. Omran, and Ahmad Salahuddin. 2022. "Evening Primrose Oil Enhances Tamoxifen's Anticancer Activity against Breast Cancer Cells by Inducing Apoptosis, Inhibiting Angiogenesis, and Arresting the Cell Cycle." *Molecules* 27 (8): 2391. https://doi.org/10.3390/molecules27082391.

Alreshoodi, Fahad M., Bassam Alsuliman, Norah M. Alotaibi, Afnan Althobaiti, Lenah E. Mukhtar, Sarah Alsaleh, Abdullah A. Alajlan, et al. 2024. "Impact of Various Washing Protocols on the Mitigation of *Escherichia coli* Contamination in Raw Salad Vegetables." *Microorganisms* 12 (10): 2103. https://doi.org/10.3390/microorganisms12102103

American Cancer Society. 2025. "American Cancer Society and ACS CAN Commends U.S. Surgeon General's Efforts to Increase Awareness and Reduce Alcohol-related Cancer." Press release, January 3, 2025. https://pressroom.cancer.org/SurgeonGeneralsAlcoholWarning.

American Cancer Society. 2026. "ACS Annual Statistics Report: Milestone 70 Percent 5-Year Survival Rate for All Cancers Combined; Largest Gains for Advanced and Fatal Cancers." Press release, January 13, 2026. Accessed April 17, 2026. https://pressroom.cancer.org/cancer-statistics-report-2026

André, Fabrice, Nofisat Ismaila, Kimberly H. Allison, William E. Barlow, Deborah E. Collyar, Senthil Damodaran, N. Lynn Henry, et al. 2022. "Biomarkers for Adjuvant Endocrine and Chemotherapy in Early-Stage Breast Cancer: ASCO Guideline Update." *Journal of Clinical Oncology* 40 (16): 1816–1837. https://doi.org/10.1200/JCO.22.00069

Armenian, Saro H., Christina Lacchetti, Ana Barac, Joseph Carver, Louis S. Constine, Neelima Denduluri, Susan Dent, et al. 2017. "Prevention and Monitoring of Cardiac Dysfunction in Survivors of Adult Cancers: American Society of Clinical Oncology Clinical Practice Guideline." *Journal of Clinical Oncology* 35 (8): 893–911. https://doi.org/10.1200/JCO.2016.70.5400

Arsic, Aleksandra, et al. 2023. "Anti-inflammatory Effect of Combining Fish Oil and Evening Primrose Oil Supplementation on Breast Cancer Patients Undergoing Chemotherapy: A Randomized Placebo-Controlled Trial." *Scientific Reports* 13:6449. https://doi.org/10.1038/s41598-023-28411-8

Barr, L., G. Metaxas, C. A. J. Harbach, L. A. Savoy, and P. D. Darbre. 2012. "Measurement of Paraben Concentrations in Human Breast Tissue at Serial Locations across the Breast from Axilla to Sternum." *Journal of Applied Toxicology* 32 (3): 219–32. https://doi.org/10.1002/jat.1786

Barroso, A., F. Estevinho, V. Hespanhol, E. Teixeira, J. Ramalho-Carvalho, and A. Araújo. 2024. "Management of Infusion-Related Reactions in Cancer Therapy: Strategies and Challenges." *ESMO Open* 9 (3): 102922. https://doi.org/10.1016/j.esmoop.2024.102922

Bedrosian, Isabelle, Mark R. Somerfield, Maria Isabel Achatz, Judy C. Boughey, Giuseppe Curigliano, Sue Friedman, Wendy K. Kohlmann, Allison W. Kurian, Christine Laronga, Filipa Lynce, Barbara S. Norquist, Jennifer K. Plichta, Patricia Rodriguez, Payal D. Shah, Marc Tischkowitz, Marie Wood, Siddhartha Yadav, Katherine Yao, and Mark E. Robson. 2024. "Germline Testing in Patients with Breast Cancer: ASCO–Society of Surgical Oncology Guideline." *Journal of Clinical Oncology* 42 (5): 584–604. https://doi.org/10.1200/JCO.23.02225

Bender, Catherine M., Susan M. Sereika, Amanda L. Gentry, Monica Wagner, Yehui Zhu, Cheryl Cuglewski, Jennie Duquette, et al. 2025. "Aerobic Exercise and Aromatase Inhibitor–Associated Musculoskeletal Symptoms: Results of a Randomized Clinical Trial." *Supportive Care in Cancer* 33 (3): 244. https://doi.org/10.1007/s00520-025-09257-4

Bidard, F.-C., A.-C. Hardy-Bessard, F. Dalenc, et al. 2022. "Switch to Fulvestrant and Palbociclib versus No Switch in Advanced Breast Cancer with Rising ESR1 Mutation during Aromatase Inhibitor and Palbociclib Therapy (PADA-1): A Randomised, Open-Label, Multicentre, Phase 3 Trial." *Lancet Oncology* 23, no. 11 (2022): 1367–77. https://doi.org/10.1016/S1470-2045(22)00555-1.

Bonaccio, Marialaura, Augusto Di Castelnuovo, Simona Costanzo, Emilia Ruggiero, Simona Esposito, Teresa Panzera, Chiara Cerletti, Maria Benedetta Donati, Giovanni de Gaetano, and Licia Iacoviello. 2024. "Mediterranean Diet Is Associated with Lower All-Cause and Cardiovascular Mortality among Long-Term Cancer Survivors." *JACC: CardioOncology* 6 (4): 602–4. https://doi.org/10.1016/j.jaccao.2024.05.012

Bone Health & Osteoporosis Foundation. 2024. "Calcium/Vitamin D Requirements, Recommended Foods & Supplements." Accessed May 15, 2026. https://www.bonehealthandosteoporosis.org/patients/treatment/calciumvitamin-d/

Bordeleau, Louise, Kathleen I. Pritchard, Charles L. Loprinzi, Marguerite Ennis, Olivia Jugovic, Doris Warr, Rola Haq, and Pamela J. Goodwin. 2010. "Multicenter, Randomized, Cross-Over Clinical Trial of Venlafaxine versus Gabapentin for the Management of Hot Flashes in Breast Cancer Survivors." *Journal of Clinical Oncology* 28 (35): 5147–5152. https://doi.org/10.1200/JCO.2010.29.9230

Boschetti, Angela, Laura Danesin, Elisa Bevilacqua, Riccardo Giada, Massimo Gion, Pierfranco Conte, and Francesca Burgio. 2025. "Investigating the Trajectories of Association Between Biomarkers and Cancer-Related Cognitive Impairment in Patients with Breast Cancer: A Systematic Review." *Cancers* 17 (21): 3522. https://doi.org/10.3390/cancers17213522

Bouvard, Véronique, Dana Loomis, Kathryn Z. Guyton, Yann Grosse, Fatiha El Ghissassi, Lamia Benbrahim-Tallaa, Neela Guha, Heidi Mattock, and Kurt Straif, on behalf of the International Agency for Research on Cancer Monograph Working Group. 2015. "Carcinogenicity of Consumption of

Red and Processed Meat." *Lancet Oncology* 16 (16): 1599–600. https://doi.org/10.1016/S1470-2045(15)00444-1

Braun, Ilana M., Kari Bohlke, Donald I. Abrams, Holly Anderson, Lynda G. Balneaves, Gil Bar-Sela, Daniel W. Bowles, et al. 2024. "Cannabis and Cannabinoids in Adults with Cancer: ASCO Guideline." *Journal of Clinical Oncology* 42 (13): 1575–1593. https://doi.org/10.1200/JCO.23.02596

Cardoso, Fatima, Laura J. van't Veer, Jan Bogaerts, Leen Slaets, Giuseppe Viale, Suzette Delaloge, Jean-Yves Pierga, et al. 2016. "70-Gene Signature as an Aid to Treatment Decisions in Early-Stage Breast Cancer." *New England Journal of Medicine* 375 (8): 717–729. https://doi.org/10.1056/NEJMoa1602253

Cardoso, Fatima, Susanne Parke, Donal J. Brennan, Paula Briggs, Gilbert Donders, Nick Panay, Nazanin Haseli-Mashhadi, et al. 2025. "Elinzanetant for Vasomotor Symptoms from Endocrine Therapy for Breast Cancer." *New England Journal of Medicine* 393 (8): 753–763. https://doi.org/10.1056/NEJMoa2415566

Carlson, Lauren E., Gordon P. Watt, Emily S. Tonorezos, Eric J. Chow, Anthony F. Yu, Meghan Woods, Charles F. Lynch, et al., for the WECARE Study Collaborative Group. 2021. "Coronary Artery Disease in Young Women after Radiation Therapy for Breast Cancer: The WECARE Study." *JACC: CardioOncology* 3 (3): 381–392. https://doi.org/10.1016/j.jaccao.2021.07.008

Castelo-Branco, C., M. Gambacciani, A. Cano, M. J. Minkin, D. Rachoń, X. Ruan, A.-M. Beer, et al. 2021. "Review & Meta-Analysis: Isopropanolic Black Cohosh Extract iCR for Menopausal Symptoms — an Update on the Evidence." *Climacteric* 24 (2): 109–119. https://doi.org/10.1080/13697137.2020.1820477

Cathey, Amber L., Vy K. Nguyen, Justin A. Colacino, Tracey J. Woodruff, Peggy Reynolds, and Max T. Aung. 2023. "Exploratory Profiles of Phenols, Parabens, and Per- and Poly-Fluoroalkyl Substances among NHANES Study Participants in Association with Previous Cancer Diagnoses." *Journal of Exposure Science and Environmental Epidemiology* 33 (5): 687–698. https://doi.org/10.1038/s41370-023-00601-6

Chen, Hai-long, Jiao-qun Zhou, Qiang Chen, and Yong-chuan Deng. 2021. "Comparison of the Sensitivity of Mammography, Ultrasound, Magnetic Resonance Imaging and Combinations of These Imaging Modalities for the Detection of Small (≤2 cm) Breast Cancer." *Medicine* 100, no. 26 (July 2, 2021): e26531. https://doi.org/10.1097/MD.0000000000026531

Collins, Karen. 2017. "HealthTalk: Flaxseed and Breast Cancer." American Institute for Cancer Research, June 6, 2017. Accessed May 18, 2026. https://www.aicr.org/resources/blog/healthtalk-flaxseed-and-breast-cancer/

Covington, Matthew F., Sophia R. O'Brien, Courtney Lawhn-Heath, Austin R. Pantel, Gary A. Ulaner, Hannah M. Linden, and Farrokh Dehdashti. 2024. "^{18}F-Labeled Fluoroestradiol PET/CT: Current Status, Gaps in Knowledge, and Controversies—AJR Expert Panel Narrative Review." *American Journal of Roentgenology* 223 (4): e2330330. https://doi.org/10.2214/AJR.23.30330.

Cuzzocrea, Marco, Rosa Di Micco, Giorgia Elisabeth Colombo, Stefania Maria Rita Rizzo, Gaetano Paone, Virginia Casati, Turki Alkhaldii, et al. 2025. "The Role of [18F]FES PET/CT in Breast Cancer Management: An Umbrella Review." *Cancers* 17 (10): 1644. https://doi.org/10.3390/cancers17101644

Daly, Grace R., Mohamad M. AlRawashdeh, John McGrath, Graham P. Dowling, Liam Cox, Sadhbh Naidoo, Darran Vareslija, Arnold D. K. Hill, and Leonie Young. 2024. "PARP Inhibitors in Breast Cancer: A Short Communication." *Current Oncology Reports* 26 (2): 103–13. https://doi.org/10.1007/s11912-023-01488-0

Davison, Zoë, Gail E. de Blacquière, Bruce R. Westley, and Felicity E. B. May. 2011. "Insulin-like Growth Factor–Dependent Proliferation and Survival of Triple-Negative Breast Cancer Cells: Implications for Therapy." *Neoplasia* 13 (6): 504–15. https://doi.org/10.1593/neo.101590

de Jager, V. D., et al. 2025. "Reporting of Molecular Test Results from Cell-

Free DNA Analyses: Expert Consensus Recommendations from the 2023 European Liquid Biopsy Society ctDNA Workshop." *eBioMedicine*. https://doi.org/10.1016/j.ebiom.2025.105123

Demos-Davies, Kimberly, Jessica Lawrence, and Davis Seelig. 2024. "Cancer Related Cognitive Impairment: A Downside of Cancer Treatment." *Frontiers in Oncology* 14:1387251. https://doi.org/10.3389/fonc.2024.1387251

Deng, Xianguang, et al. 2023. "Updating the Therapeutic Role of Ginsenosides in Breast Cancer: A Bibliometrics Study to an In-Depth Review." Frontiers in Pharmacology 14:1226629. https://doi.org/10.3389/fphar.2023.1226629

Dobovišek, Luka, Simona Borštnar, Nataša Debeljak, and Simona Kranjc Brezar. 2024. "Cannabinoids and Triple-Negative Breast Cancer Treatment." *Frontiers in Immunology* 15. https://doi.org/10.3389/fimmu.2024.1386548

Dodson, Robin E., Marcia Nishioka, Laurel J. Standley, Laura J. Perovich, Julia Green Brody, and Ruthann A. Rudel. 2012. "Endocrine Disruptors and Asthma-Associated Chemicals in Consumer Products." *Environmental Health Perspectives* 120 (7): 935–943. https://doi.org/10.1289/ehp.1104052

Downs, Craig A., Mohammad Mehdi Amin, Maryam Tabatabaeian, Afsane Chavoshani, Elham Amjadi, Alireza Afshari, and Roya Kelishadi. 2023. "Parabens Preferentially Accumulate in Metastatic Breast Tumors Compared to Benign Breast Tumors and the Association of Breast Cancer Risk Factors with Paraben Accumulation." *Environmental Advances* 11: 100325. https://doi.org/10.1016/j.envadv.2022.100325.

Early Breast Cancer Trialists' Collaborative Group (EBCTCG). 2015. "Adjuvant Bisphosphonate Treatment in Early Breast Cancer: Meta-Analyses of Individual Patient Data from Randomised Trials." *The Lancet* 386 (10001): 1353–1361. https://doi.org/10.1016/S0140-6736(15)60908-4

ecancer. 2024. "Ten-Year Study Shows Tomosynthesis Improves Breast Cancer Detection." September 18, 2024. https://ecancer.org/en/news/25340-ten-year-study-shows-tomosynthesis-improves-breast-cancer-detection

Ellison, Gary L., Kathy J. Helzlsouer, Sonia M. Rosenfield, Yun Kim, Rebecca L. Ashare, Anne H. Blaes, Jennifer Cullen, et al. 2024. "Perceptions,

Prevalence, and Patterns of Cannabis Use Among Cancer Patients Treated at 12 NCI-Designated Cancer Centers." *Journal of the National Cancer Institute Monographs* 2024 (66): 202–217. https://doi.org/10.1093/jncimonographs/lgae029

Faubion, Stephanie S., Lisa C. Larkin, Cynthia A. Stuenkel, Gloria A. Bachmann, Lisa A. Chism, Risa Kagan, Andrew M. Kaunitz, et al. 2018. "Management of Genitourinary Syndrome of Menopause in Women with or at High Risk for Breast Cancer: Consensus Recommendations from The North American Menopause Society and The International Society for the Study of Women's Sexual Health." *Menopause* 25 (6): 596–608. https://doi.org/10.1097/GME.0000000000001121

Fornell, Dave. 2024. "90% of Breast Imaging Centers Now Offer 3D Tomosynthesis." Radiology Business, August 5, 2024. https://radiologybusiness.com/topics/medical-imaging/womens-imaging/breast-imaging/90-breast-imaging-centers-now-offer-3d-tomosynthesis

Fritz, Heidi, Dugald Seely, Gillian Flower, Becky Skidmore, Rochelle Fernandes, Sarah Vadeboncoeur, Deborah Kennedy, et al. 2013. "Soy, Red Clover, and Isoflavones and Breast Cancer: A Systematic Review." *PLOS ONE* 8 (11): e81968. https://doi.org/10.1371/journal.pone.0081968

Fritz, Heidi, Dugald Seely, Jessie McGowan, Becky Skidmore, Rochelle Fernandes, Deborah A. Kennedy, Kieran Cooley, et al. 2014. "Black Cohosh and Breast Cancer: A Systematic Review." *Integrative Cancer Therapies* 13 (1): 12–29. https://doi.org/10.1177/1534735413477191.

Fusco, Nicola, et al. 2025. "International Society of Liquid Biopsy (ISLB) Perspective on Minimal Requirements for ctDNA Testing in Solid Tumors." *Journal of Liquid Biopsy*. https://doi.org/10.1016/j.jlb.2025.100317

Glynne, Sarah, Daniel Reisel, Aini Kamal, and Louise Newson. 2025. "Patient Experience of Menopause Care after Breast Cancer in the UK: A Cross-Sectional Study." *Menopause* 32 (5): 396–408. https://doi.org/10.1097/GME.0000000000002504

Goñi-Arana, Ane, Jorge Pérez-Martín, and Francisco Javier Díez. 2024. "Breast Thermography: A Systematic Review and Meta-Analysis." *Systematic Reviews* 13 (1): 295. https://doi.org/10.1186/s13643-024-02708-9.

Grand View Research. 2025. "U.S. Dietary Supplements Market (2026–2033) Size, Share & Trends Analysis Report." Accessed May 18, 2026. https://www.grandviewresearch.com/industry-analysis/us-dietary-supplements-market-report

Grant, William B., Sunil J. Wimalawansa, Pawel Pludowski, and Richard Z. Cheng. 2025. "Vitamin D: Evidence-Based Health Benefits and Recommendations for Population Guidelines." *Nutrients* 17, no. 2: 277. https://doi.org/10.3390/nu17020277

Gullett, Joseph M., Ronald A. Cohen, Gee-Su Yang, Virginia S. Menzies, Robert A. Fieo, Debra L. Kelly, Angela R. Starkweather, Colleen Jackson-Cook, and Debra E. Lyon. 2019. "Relationship of Fatigue with Cognitive Performance in Women with Early-Stage Breast Cancer over 2 Years." *Psycho-Oncology* 28 (5): 997–1003. https://doi.org/10.1002/pon.5028

Hajirahimkhan, Afsaneh, et al. 2023. "Breast Cancer Prevention with Liquiritigenin from Licorice through the Inhibition of Aromatase and Protein Biosynthesis in High-Risk Women's Breast Tissue." *Scientific Reports* 13:8734. https://doi.org/10.1038/s41598-023-34762-z

Hong, Catherine H. L., Joel J. Napeñas, Brian D. Hodgson, Monique A. Stokman, Vickie Mathers-Stauffer, Linda S. Elting, Fred K. L. Spijkervet, and Michael T. Brennan. 2010. "A Systematic Review of Dental Disease in Patients Undergoing Cancer Therapy." *Supportive Care in Cancer* 18 (8): 1007–21. https://doi.org/10.1007/s00520-010-0873-2

Huang, Yi-Ran, Hua-Qing Xing, Yi-Ran Yan, Yu-Cheng Wang, Yuan Feng, Robert D. Smith, Zhaohui Su, et al. 2026. "Quality of Life in Breast Cancer Survivors: A Meta-Analysis of Case-Control Studies." *Psycho-Oncology*. Published ahead of print, February 18, 2026. https://doi.org/10.1002/pon.70398

Hung, Chen-Sin, Yi-Ting Cheng, Ruei-Hong Li, Charles H. Hillman, Neha P. Gothe, Feng-Tzu Chen, Hsing-Jung Yeh, Fei-Fei Ren, and Yu-Kai Chang. 2025. "Effect of Exercise Interventions on Cognitive Function in Breast Cancer Patients and Survivors: A Systematic Review with Meta-Analysis." *Breast Cancer* 32 (6): 1180–1196. https://doi.org/10.1007/s12282-025-01757-9.

Hunter, N. B., H. A. Parsons, L. Cope, et al. 2026. "The Pathologic Response Evaluation and Detection in Circulating Tumor-DNA Study: Ultrasensitive Circulating Tumor-DNA Assessment of Breast Cancer Minimal Residual Disease." *Journal of Clinical Oncology*. https://doi.org/10.1200/JCO-25-02934

International Agency for Research on Cancer. 2012. *Chemical Agents and Related Occupations*. IARC Monographs on the Evaluation of Carcinogenic Risks to Humans, vol. 100F. Lyon: IARC. https://publications.iarc.who.int/Book-And-Report-Series/Iarc-Monographs-On-The-Identification-Of-Carcinogenic-Hazards-To-Humans/Chemical-Agents-And-Related-Occupations-2012

International Agency for Research on Cancer. 2025. "Alcohol: A Major Preventable Cause of Cancer." Press release no. 371, October 8, 2025. https://www.iarc.who.int/wp-content/uploads/2025/10/pr371_E.pdf

International Agency for Research on Cancer. 2025. *Perfluorooctanoic Acid (PFOA) and Perfluorooctanesulfonic Acid (PFOS)*. IARC Monographs on the Identification of Carcinogenic Hazards to Humans, vol. 135. Lyon: IARC. https://publications.iarc.who.int/Book-And-Report-Series/Iarc-Monographs-On-The-Identification-Of-Carcinogenic-Hazards-To-Humans/Perfluorooctanoic-Acid-PFOA-And-Perfluorooctanesulfonic-Acid-PFOS--2025

Jarry, H., Sabine Leonhardt, C. Gorkow, and W. Wuttke. 1994. "In Vitro Prolactin but Not LH and FSH Release Is Inhibited by Compounds in Extracts of *Agnus castus*: Direct Evidence for a Dopaminergic Principle by the Dopamine Receptor Assay." *Experimental and Clinical Endocrinology & Diabetes* 102 (6): 448–54. https://doi.org/10.1055/s-0029-1211317.

Johns, Claire, Susan M. Seav, Sally A. Dominick, Jessica R. Gorman, Hongying Li, Loki Natarajan, Jun James Mao, and H. Irene Su. 2016. "Informing Hot Flash Treatment Decisions for Breast Cancer Survivors: A Systematic Review of Randomized Trials Comparing Active Interventions." *Breast Cancer Research and Treatment* 156 (3): 415–426. https://doi.org/10.1007/s10549-016-3765-4

Johnson, Rebecca H., Ashley Speckhart, Franklin Chien, and Archie Bleyer. 2025. "Emerging Evidence Links Cannabis Use to Increased Risk of Breast and Testicular Cancer in Young Americans." *Academia Oncology* 2 (2). https://doi.org/10.20935/AcadOnco7758

Kahl, Kristie L. 2026. "ctDNA in Early-Stage Breast Cancer: Prognostic Power vs Clinical Actionability." *OncLive*, May 13, 2026. https://www.onclive.com/view/ctdna-in-early-stage-breast-cancer-prognostic-power-vs-clinical-actionability

Kalinsky, Kevin, Judy E. Garber, Joseph A. Sparano, Zhimin Shao, Fei Xu, Alvaro Ruiz, Mikhail Druker, et al. 2021. "21-Gene Assay to Inform Chemotherapy Benefit in Node-Positive Breast Cancer." *New England Journal of Medicine* 385 (25): 2336–2347. https://doi.org/10.1056/NEJMoa2108873

Kasprzak, Aldona. 2021. "Insulin-Like Growth Factor 1 (IGF-1) Signaling in Glucose Metabolism in Colorectal Cancer." *International Journal of Molecular Sciences* 22 (12): 6434. https://doi.org/10.3390/ijms22126434.

Kirshner, Jeffrey J., Maxwell C. McDonald III, Flavio Kruter, Andrew S. Guinigundo, Linda Vanni, Cathy L. Maxwell, Maureen Reiner, Terry E. Upchurch, Jacob Garcia, and Phuong Khanh Morrow. 2018. "NOLAN: A Randomized, Phase 2 Study to Estimate the Effect of Prophylactic Naproxen or Loratadine vs No Prophylactic Treatment on Bone Pain in Patients with Early-Stage Breast Cancer Receiving Chemotherapy and Pegfilgrastim." *Supportive Care in Cancer* 26 (4): 1323–34. https://doi.org/10.1007/s00520-017-3959-2

Klenske, Nick. 2025. "Contrast-Enhanced Mammography as an Alternative to MRI." *RSNA News*, October 20, 2025. https://www.rsna.org/news/2025/october/cem-alternative-to-mri-breast-screening

Ko, Gordon D., Nadia B. Nowacki, Leigh Arseneau, Michelle Eitel, and Andrea Hum. 2010. "Omega-3 Fatty Acids for Neuropathic Pain: Case Series." *Clinical Journal of Pain* 26, no. 2: 168–72. https://doi.org/10.1097/AJP.0b013e3181bb8533

Kotsopoulos, Joanne, Marta Seca, Jacek Gronwald, Tomasz Huzarski, Pål Møller, Raymond H. Kim, Christian F. Singer, et al. 2025. "Menopausal Hormone Therapy and the Risk of Breast Cancer in Women with a Pathogenic Variant in *BRCA1* or *BRCA2*." *JNCI: Journal of the National Cancer Institute* 118 (5): 856–64. https://doi.org/10.1093/jnci/djaf363

Kulkarni, Swati, et al. 2025. "A Large-Scale Multicenter Phase II Study Evaluating the Protective Effect of a Tissue Selective Estrogen Complex (TSEC) in Women with Newly Diagnosed Ductal Carcinoma in Situ." Paper presented at the American Society of Clinical Oncology Annual Meeting, Chicago, IL, June 1, 2025. Abstract 512.

Kwan, Marilyn L., Lawrence H. Kushi, Erin Weltzien, Emily K. Tam, Adrienne Castillo, Carol Sweeney, and Bette J. Caan. 2010. "Alcohol Consumption and Breast Cancer Recurrence and Survival Among Women With Early-Stage Breast Cancer: The Life After Cancer Epidemiology Study." *Journal of Clinical Oncology* 28 (29): 4410–4416. https://doi.org/10.1200/JCO.2010.29.2730.

Kwan, Marilyn L., Wendy Y. Chen, Shirley W. Flatt, Erin K. Weltzien, Sarah J. Nechuta, Elizabeth M. Poole, Michelle D. Holmes, Ruth E. Patterson, Xiao Ou Shu, John P. Pierce, and Bette J. Caan. 2013. "Postdiagnosis Alcohol Consumption and Breast Cancer Prognosis in the After Breast Cancer Pooling Project." *Cancer Epidemiology, Biomarkers & Prevention* 22 (1): 32–41. https://doi.org/10.1158/1055-9965.EPI-12-1022.

Kwan, Marilyn L., Emily Valice, Isaac J. Ergas, Janise M. Roh, Bette J. Caan, Elizabeth M. Cespedes Feliciano, Tatjana Kolevska, Terryl J. Hartman, Charles P. Quesenberry Jr., Christine B. Ambrosone, and Lawrence H.

Kushi. 2023. "Alcohol Consumption and Prognosis and Survival in Breast Cancer Survivors: The Pathways Study." *Cancer* 129 (24): 3938–51. https://doi.org/10.1002/cncr.34972

Kyo, Satoru, Noriyoshi Ishikawa, Kohei Nakamura, and Kentaro Nakayama. 2020. "The Fallopian Tube as Origin of Ovarian Cancer: Change of Diagnostic and Preventive Strategies." *Cancer Medicine* 9 (2): 421–431. https://doi.org/10.1002/cam4.2725

Law, Jennifer H., Golareh Habibi, Kaiji Hu, Hamid Masoudi, Michelle Y. C. Wang, Anna L. Stratford, Eugene Park, et al. 2008. "Phosphorylated Insulin-Like Growth Factor-I/Insulin Receptor Is Present in All Breast Cancer Subtypes and Is Related to Poor Survival." *Cancer Research* 68 (24): 10238–46. https://doi.org/10.1158/0008-5472.CAN-08-2755

Lederman, Samuel, Faith D. Ottery, Antonio Cano, Nanette Santoro, Marla Shapiro, Petra Stute, Rebecca C. Thurston, et al. 2023. "Fezolinetant for Treatment of Moderate-to-Severe Vasomotor Symptoms Associated with Menopause (SKYLIGHT 1): A Phase 3 Randomised Controlled Study." *The Lancet* 401 (10382): 1091–1102. https://doi.org/10.1016/S0140-6736(23)00085-5

Lee, YoungJoo, YoungRan Jin, WonChung Lim, SangMi Ji, Songho Choi, Siyoul Jang, and SeungKi Lee. 2003. "A Ginsenoside-Rh1, a Component of Ginseng Saponin, Activates Estrogen Receptor in Human Breast Carcinoma MCF-7 Cells." *Journal of Steroid Biochemistry and Molecular Biology* 84 (4): 463–468. https://doi.org/10.1016/S0960-0760(03)00067-0

Lewin, John, and Maxine Jochelson. 2017. "Contrast Enhanced Digital Mammography." White paper, Society of Breast Imaging, May 1, 2017. https://www.sbi-online.org/white-papers/contrast-enhanced-digital-mammography

Liu, J., J. E. Burdette, H. Xu, C. Gu, R. B. van Breemen, K. P. L. Bhat, N. Booth, et al. 2001. "Evaluation of Estrogenic Activity of Plant Extracts for the Potential Treatment of Menopausal Symptoms." *Journal of Agricultural and Food Chemistry* 49 (5): 2472–2479. https://doi.org/10.1021/jf0014157

Loprinzi, Charles L., John W. Kugler, Jeff A. Sloan, James A. Mailliard, Brigitte I. LaVasseur, Debra L. Barton, Paul J. Novotny, et al. 2000. "Venlafaxine in Management of Hot Flashes in Survivors of Breast Cancer: A Randomised Controlled Trial." *The Lancet* 356 (9247): 2059–2063. https://doi.org/10.1016/S0140-6736(00)03403-6

Makarem, Nour, Elisa V. Bandera, Yong Lin, Paul F. Jacques, Richard B. Hayes, and Niyati Parekh. 2018. "Consumption of Sugars, Sugary Foods, and Sugary Beverages in Relation to Adiposity-Related Cancer Risk in the Framingham Offspring Cohort (1991–2013)." *Cancer Prevention Research* 11 (6): 347–58. https://doi.org/10.1158/1940-6207.CAPR-17-0218

Mannel, Marcus. 2004. "Drug Interactions with St John's Wort: Mechanisms and Clinical Implications." *Drug Safety* 27 (11): 773–797. https://doi.org/10.2165/00002018-200427110-00003

Mao, Jun James, Mary A. Bowman, Sharon X. Xie, Deborah Bruner, Angela DeMichele, and John T. Farrar. 2015. "Electroacupuncture versus Gabapentin for Hot Flashes among Breast Cancer Survivors: A Randomized Placebo-Controlled Trial." *Journal of Clinical Oncology* 33 (31): 3615–3620. https://doi.org/10.1200/JCO.2015.60.9412

Mathijssen, Ron H. J., Jaap Verweij, Peter de Bruijn, Walter J. Loos, and Alex Sparreboom. 2002. "Effects of St. John's Wort on Irinotecan Metabolism." *JNCI: Journal of the National Cancer Institute* 94 (16): 1247–1249. https://doi.org/10.1093/jnci/94.16.1247

McKay, C., T. Rahman, B. Ghimire, and M. Girgis. 2026. "Circulating Tumor DNA in Breast Cancer: Diagnostic Insights From a Case Series." *Cureus* 18 (1): e100833. https://doi.org/10.7759/cureus.100833

McRorie, Johnson W., Maria E. Petrey, Kyle J. Sloan, and Roger Gibb. 2021. "S190 Docusate Is Not Different from Placebo for Stool Softening: A Comprehensive Review." *American Journal of Gastroenterology* 116 (S1): S85. https://doi.org/10.14309/01.ajg.0000773232.60122.be

Memorial Sloan Kettering Cancer Center. 2022. "Evening Primrose Oil." Last updated February 16, 2022. Accessed May 18, 2026. https://www.mskcc.org/cancer-care/integrative-medicine/herbs/evening-primrose-oil

Memorial Sloan Kettering Cancer Center, 2022. "Wild Yam: Purported Benefits, Side Effects and More." July 12th. https://www.mskcc.org/cancer-care/integrative-medicine/herbs/wild-yam

Morin, Charles M., Célyne Bastien, Bernard Guay, Monelly Radouco-Thomas, Jacinthe Leblanc, and Annie Vallières. 2004. "Randomized Clinical Trial of Supervised Tapering and Cognitive Behavior Therapy to Facilitate Benzodiazepine Discontinuation in Older Adults with Chronic Insomnia." *American Journal of Psychiatry* 161 (2): 332–342. https://doi.org/10.1176/appi.ajp.161.2.332

Muhamad, Razaq, Argyro Akrivaki, Georgia Papagiannopoulou, Panagiotis Zavridis, and Panagiotis Zis. 2023. "The Role of Vitamin B6 in Peripheral Neuropathy: A Systematic Review." *Nutrients* 15, no. 13: 2823. https://doi.org/10.3390/nu15132823

Nakajima, Erika, Lena Nguyen, Ning Liu, Danielle Rodin, Eitan Amir, Peter C. Austin, Paaladinesh Thavendiranathan, and Husam Abdel-Qadir. 2026. "Long-Term Risk of Cardiovascular Disease after Contemporary Left-Sided Breast Radiation Therapy." *JAMA Network Open* 9 (4): e264098. https://doi.org/10.1001/jamanetworkopen.2026.4098

National Comprehensive Cancer Network (NCCN). n.d. "Detection, Prevention, and Risk Reduction." NCCN Clinical Practice Guidelines in Oncology. Accessed May 4, 2026. https://www.nccn.org/guidelines/category_2

National Comprehensive Cancer Network (NCCN). 2025. *NCCN Clinical Practice Guidelines in Oncology: Ovarian Cancer, Including Fallopian Tube Cancer and Primary Peritoneal Cancer.* Version 3.2025. Plymouth Meeting, PA: National Comprehensive Cancer Network. July 16, 2025. Accessed May 4, 2026. https://www.nccn.org/professionals/physician_gls/pdf/ovarian.pdf

National Comprehensive Cancer Network (NCCN). 2025. *NCCN Guidelines for Patients: Genetic Testing for Hereditary Breast, Ovarian, Pancreatic, and Prostate Cancer.* Plymouth Meeting, PA: National Comprehensive

Cancer Network. Accessed May 4, 2026. https://www.nccn.org/patients/guidelines/content/PDF/genetics-patient.pdf

Negrão, Luís, Pedro Almeida, Sérgio Alcino, Helena Duro, Teresa Libório, Ulisses Melo Silva, Ricardo Figueira, Sílvia Gonçalves, and Laura Neto Parra. 2014. "Effect of the Combination of Uridine Nucleotides, Folic Acid and Vitamin B12 on the Clinical Expression of Peripheral Neuropathies." *Pain Management* 4, no. 3: 191–96. https://doi.org/10.2217/pmt.14.10

Noordhoek, Iris, Kai Treuner, Hein Putter, Yi Zhang, Jenna Wong, Elma Meershoek-Klein Kranenbarg, Marjolijn Duijm-de Carpentier, Cornelis J. H. van de Velde, Catherine A. Schnabel, and Gerrit-Jan Liefers. 2021. "Breast Cancer Index Predicts Extended Endocrine Benefit to Individualize Selection of Patients with HR+ Early-Stage Breast Cancer for 10 Years of Endocrine Therapy." *Clinical Cancer Research* 27 (1): 311–319. https://doi.org/10.1158/1078-0432.CCR-20-2737

Nyrop, Kirsten A., Leigh F. Callahan, Rebecca J. Cleveland, Liubov L. Arbeeva, Betsy S. Hackney, and Hyman B. Muss. 2017. "Randomized Controlled Trial of a Home-Based Walking Program to Reduce Moderate to Severe Aromatase Inhibitor-Associated Arthralgia in Breast Cancer Survivors." *The Oncologist* 22 (10): 1238–1249. https://doi.org/10.1634/theoncologist.2017-0174

Office of Dietary Supplements, National Institutes of Health. n.d. "Dietary Supplement Health and Education Act of 1994." Accessed May 18, 2026. https://ods.od.nih.gov/About/DSHEA_Wording.aspx

Oldacres, Laura, Josephine Hegarty, Patricia O'Regan, Noreen M. Murphy-Coakley, and Mohamad M. Saab. 2022. "Interventions Promoting Cognitive Function in Patients Experiencing Cancer Related Cognitive Impairment: A Systematic Review." *Psycho-Oncology*. Published ahead of print, November 28, 2022. https://doi.org/10.1002/pon.6073

O'Malley, David M., Thomas C. Krivak, Nashwa Kabil, Jiefen Munley, and Kathleen N. Moore. 2023. "PARP Inhibitors in Ovarian Cancer: A Review." *Target Oncology* 18 (4): 471–503. https://doi.org/10.1007/s11523-023-00970-w

Pandya, Kishan J., Gary R. Morrow, Joseph A. Roscoe, Honghong Zhao, Jane T. Hickok, Ernest Pajon, Thomas J. Sweeney, Tapas K. Banerjee, and Patrick J. Flynn. 2005. "Gabapentin for Hot Flashes in 420 Women with Breast Cancer: A Randomised Double-Blind Placebo-Controlled Trial." *The Lancet* 366 (9488): 818–824. https://doi.org/10.1016/S0140-6736(05)67215-7

Park, Mi Kyung, Hyeok Yi Kwon, Woong Shick Ahn, Sunghee Bae, Mi Ran Rhyu, and Yong Jin Lee. 2009. "Estrogen Activities and the Cellular Effects of Natural Progesterone from Wild Yam Extract in MCF-7 Human Breast Cancer Cells." *American Journal of Chinese Medicine* 37 (1): 159–67. https://doi.org/10.1142/S0192415X09006746.

Parsons, H. A., et al. 2026. "Tumor-Informed Circulating Tumor DNA Analysis to Assess Molecular Residual Disease for Prognosis and Prediction of Benefit from Palbociclib in the PALLAS Trial." Abstract RF3-04. Presented at the 2025 San Antonio Breast Cancer Symposium, San Antonio, TX, December 9–12, 2025. *Clinical Cancer Research* 32 (4 Supplement): RF3-04. https://doi.org/10.1158/1557-3265.SABCS25-RF3-04

Patel, Bhavika K., Molly B. Carnahan, and Donald Northfelt, et al. 2024. "Prospective Study of Supplemental Screening With Contrast-Enhanced Mammography in Women With Elevated Risk of Breast Cancer: Results of the Prevalence Round." *Journal of Clinical Oncology* 42, no. 32 (July 26, 2024). https://doi.org/10.1200/JCO.22.02819

Piccart, Martine, Marion Procter, Debora Fumagalli, Evandro de Azambuja, Emma Clark, Michael S. Ewer, Eleonora Restuccia, et al. 2021. "Adjuvant Pertuzumab and Trastuzumab in Early HER2-Positive Breast Cancer in the APHINITY Trial: 6 Years' Follow-Up." *Journal of Clinical Oncology* 39 (13): 1448–57. https://doi.org/10.1200/JCO.20.01204.

Powles, Trevor J., Anthony Howell, D. Gareth Evans, Eugene V. McCloskey, Sue Ashley, Rosemary Greenhalgh, Jenny Affen, Lesley Ann Flook, and Alwynne Tidy. 2008. "Red Clover Isoflavones Are Safe and Well Tolerated in Women with a Family History of Breast Cancer." *Menopause International* 14 (1): 6–12. https://doi.org/10.1258/mi.2007.007033

Putz, Zsuzsanna, Dóra Tordai, Noémi Hajdú, Orsolya Erzsébet Vági, Miklós Kempler, Magdolna Békeffy, Anna Erzsébet Körei, et al. 2022. "Vitamin D in the Prevention and Treatment of Diabetic Neuropathy." *Clinical Therapeutics* 44, no. 5: 813–23. https://doi.org/10.1016/j.clinthera.2022.03.012

Siegel, Rebecca L., Tyler B. Kratzer, Nikita S. Wagle, Hyuna Sung, and Ahmedin Jemal. 2026. "Cancer Statistics, 2026." *CA: A Cancer Journal for Clinicians* 46 (1): e70043. https://doi.org/10.3322/caac.70043

Snellings, Robin, Takahiro Matsuo, Sebastian Wurster, Ying Jiang, Jeffery Tarrand, Sung-Yeon Cho, and Dimitrios P. Kontoyiannis. 2025. "P-2294. Listeriosis in Cancer Patients: Uncommon and Protean." *Open Forum Infectious Diseases* 12 (Supplement 1): ofae631.2447. https://doi.org/10.1093/ofid/ofae631.2447

Sparano, Joseph A., Robert J. Gray, Della F. Makower, Kathleen I. Pritchard, Kathy S. Albain, Daniel F. Hayes, Charles E. Geyer, et al. 2018. "Adjuvant Chemotherapy Guided by a 21-Gene Expression Assay in Breast Cancer." *New England Journal of Medicine* 379 (2): 111–121. https://doi.org/10.1056/NEJMoa1804710

Skaznik-Wikiel, Malgorzata E., et al. 2018. "Radical Trachelectomy for Early-Stage Cervical Cancer: Oncologic and Obstetric Outcomes." *Journal of Gynecologic Oncology* 29 (3): e37. https://doi.org/10.3802/jgo.2018.29.e37

Taha, Tarek, David Meiri, Samira Talhamy, Mira Wollner, Avivit Peer, and Gil Bar-Sela. 2019. "Cannabis Impacts Tumor Response Rate to Nivolumab in Patients with Advanced Malignancies." *The Oncologist* 24 (4): 549–554. https://doi.org/10.1634/theoncologist.2018-0383

Tamir, S., M. Eizenberg, D. Somjen, N. Stern, R. Shelach, A. Kaye, and J. Vaya. 2000. "Estrogenic and Antiproliferative Properties of Glabridin from Licorice in Human Breast Cancer Cells." *Cancer Research* 60 (20): 5704–5709. https://pubmed.ncbi.nlm.nih.gov/11059763/

Tew, William P., Christina Lacchetti, Amanda Ellis, Katie Maxian, Susana Banerjee, Michael Bookman, Melissa B. Jones, et al. 2020. "PARP

Inhibitors in the Management of Ovarian Cancer: ASCO Guideline." *Journal of Clinical Oncology* 38 (30): 3468–93. https://doi.org/10.1200/JCO.20.01924

Treasure, Michelle, Alicia Thomas, Stephen Ganocy, Augustine Hong, Smitha S. Krishnamurthi, David L. Bajor, Nathan A. Berger, and Neal J. Meropol. 2021. "A Pilot Study of a Low Glycemic Load Diet in Patients with Stage I–III Colorectal Cancer." *Journal of Gastrointestinal Oncology* 12 (3): 910–20. https://doi.org/10.21037/jgo-20-330

Tutt, Andrew N. J., Judy E. Garber, Bella Kaufman, Giuseppe Viale, Debora Fumagalli, Priya Rastogi, Richard D. Gelber, et al. 2021. "Adjuvant Olaparib for Patients with BRCA1- or BRCA2-Mutated Breast Cancer." New England Journal of Medicine 384 (25): 2394–2405. https://doi.org/10.1056/NEJMoa2105215.

U.S. Food and Drug Administration. 2021. "Breast Cancer Screening: Thermogram No Substitute for Mammogram." January 13, 2021. https://www.fda.gov/consumers/consumer-updates/breast-cancer-screening-thermogram-no-substitute-mammogram

Vallianou, N., A. Evangelopoulos, and P. Koutalas. 2009. "Alpha-Lipoic Acid and Diabetic Neuropathy." *Review of Diabetic Studies* 6, no. 4: 230–36. https://doi.org/10.1900/RDS.2009.6.230

van Die, M. Diana, Kerry M. Bone, Kala Visvanathan, Cecile Kyrø, Dagfinn Aune, Carolyn Ee, and Channing J. Paller. 2024. "Phytonutrients and Outcomes Following Breast Cancer: A Systematic Review and Meta-Analysis of Observational Studies." *JNCI Cancer Spectrum* 8 (1): pkad104. https://doi.org/10.1093/jncics/pkad104

Weil, Andrew, MD. 2012. "Is Evening Primrose Oil Safe After Breast Cancer?" May 8. https://www.drweil.com/vitamins-supplements-herbs/supplements-remedies/is-evening-primrose-oil-safe-after-breast-cancer/

Weiss, Marisa C., Julianne E. Hibbs, Meghan E. Buckley, Sherry R. Danese, Adam Leitenberger, Melissa Bollmann-Jenkins, Sam W. Meske, et al. 2022. "A Coala-T-Cannabis Survey Study of Breast Cancer Patients'

Use of Cannabis before, during, and after Treatment." *Cancer* 128 (1): 160–168. https://doi.org/10.1002/cncr.33906

Winkler, Juliane, Pengyuan Liu, Kiet Phong, Johanna H. Hinrichs, Nassim Ataii, Katherine Williams, Elin Hadler-Olsen, et al. 2022. "Bisphenol A Replacement Chemicals, BPF and BPS, Induce Protumorigenic Changes in Human Mammary Gland Organoid Morphology and Proteome." *Proceedings of the National Academy of Sciences* 119 (11): e2115308119. https://doi.org/10.1073/pnas.2115308119

Winschel, Timothy R., Kellie Weinhold, Patrick M. Schnell, Stephanie Gorka, Maryam Lustberg, Darrin Aase, Zihan Melink, et al. 2025. "The Association of the MIND Diet and Its Components with Cognitive Function in Postmenopausal Breast Cancer Survivors." *Supportive Care in Cancer* 33 (8): 736. https://doi.org/10.1007/s00520-025-09789-9

World Health Organization Regional Office for Europe. 2023. "No Level of Alcohol Consumption Is Safe for Our Health." January 4, 2023. https://www.who.int/europe/news/item/04-01-2023-no-level-of-alcohol-consumption-is-safe-for-our-health

Worster, Brooke, Emily R. Hajjar, and Nathan Handley. 2022. "Cannabis Use in Patients with Cancer: A Clinical Review." *JCO Oncology Practice* 18 (11): 743–749. https://doi.org/10.1200/OP.22.00080

Yeh, Eren D., et al. 2025. "ACR Appropriateness Criteria® Female Breast Cancer Screening: 2025 Update." *Journal of the American College of Radiology* 22, no. 11 (November 2025): S508–S530

Yeo, Chang Dong, Young Ae Kim, Hwa Young Lee, Jin Woo Kim, Sang Haak Lee, Seung Joon Kim, Soon Seog Kwon, Yong Hyun Kim, and Seok Chan Kim. 2017. "Inhibiting IGF-1R Attenuates Cell Proliferation and VEGF Production in IGF-1R Over-Expressing EGFR Mutant Non-Small Cell Lung Cancer Cells." *Experimental Lung Research* 43 (1): 29–37. https://doi.org/10.1080/01902148.2017.1282994

Yue, Grace Gar-Lee, Lok-Sze Wong, Hoi-Wing Leung, Si Gao, Julia Yuen-Shan Tsang, Zhi-Xiu Lin, Bonita Ka-Bo Law, Gary Man-Kit Tse, and Clara Bik-San Lau. 2019. "Is Danggui Safe to be Taken by Breast Cancer Patients?—A Skepticism Finally Answered by Comprehensive Preclinical Evidence." *Frontiers in Pharmacology* 10 (June): article 706. https://doi.org/10.3389/fphar.2019.00706

Zhang, Juan, Jie Chen, Boni Ding, Yongping Liang, Kai Liu, Ling Wang, Yuan Le, et al. 2022. "Probiotic Supplement Attenuates Chemotherapy-Related Cognitive Impairment in Patients with Breast Cancer: A Randomised, Double-Blind, and Placebo-Controlled Trial." *European Journal of Cancer* 161: 10–22. https://doi.org/10.1016/j.ejca.2021.11.006.

Zhang, Y., G. Li, S. Zhang, Y. Zhou, Y. Lv, L. Feng, and L. Yu. 2025. "Effects of Exercise on Depression and Anxiety in Breast Cancer Survivors: A Systematic Review and Meta-Analysis of Randomized Controlled Trials." *Cancer Medicine* 14: e70671. https://doi.org/10.1002/cam4.70671.

About the Author

Dr. Tiffany Troso-Sandoval, MD, is a board-certified medical oncologist, physician guide, and fierce advocate for women navigating cancer. Trained at Princeton, Cornell Medical College, and Memorial Sloan Kettering Cancer Center, she spent more than twenty-five years at the forefront of breast and gynecologic oncology, caring for thousands of women in their most vulnerable moments.

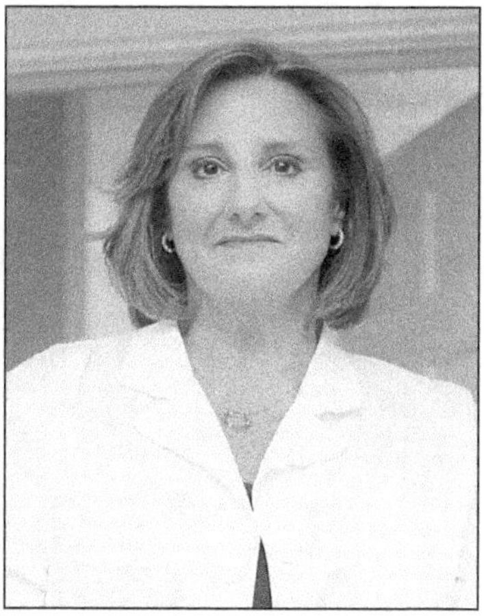

Then her own life brought her to a crossroads. Facing a serious health challenge of her own, she stepped away from full-time clinical practice, carrying a truth she could no longer set aside. That receiving treatment and truly navigating cancer care are not the same thing. It was the knowledge that changed everything.

From that reckoning was born *Winning the Cancer Journey*, her patient education platform and life's mission. Through it, she has guided high-functioning women to step out of the passive patient role the medical system creates and into their power as the true CEO of their own cancer care.

Today, Dr. Troso-Sandoval reaches women across the country through her *Empowered Patient Method*, *The Empowered Cancer Patient* podcast, and her consulting practice, Second Look Oncology. She has built a community of women who no longer sit silently in the exam room, hoping someone will explain what they need to know. They walk in prepared, self-advocating, and in control.

This book is her most complete offering yet: the one she wishes every woman had in her hands from the moment of diagnosis. It is written for the woman who will not accept confusion as a condition of survival.

www.ingramcontent.com/pod-product-compliance
Lightning Source LLC
LaVergne TN
LVHW050800061126
851857LV00012B/622
* 9 7 8 1 9 7 1 2 8 8 0 8 6 *